Fit Body Fit Mind
Your Practical Guide to Aging Well

Lawrence S. Richardson, Jr.

International Sports Sciences Association
Certified Senior Fitness Specialist

Visit our companion website, <u>Xeniors.com,</u> for free exercise videos & the latest fitness information.

DEDICATION

This book is dedicated to my mother, Lee Richardson, who taught me fitness – achieved through consistent, non-destructive exercise, a healthy diet, and challenging the mind -- is the key to a fulfilling life.

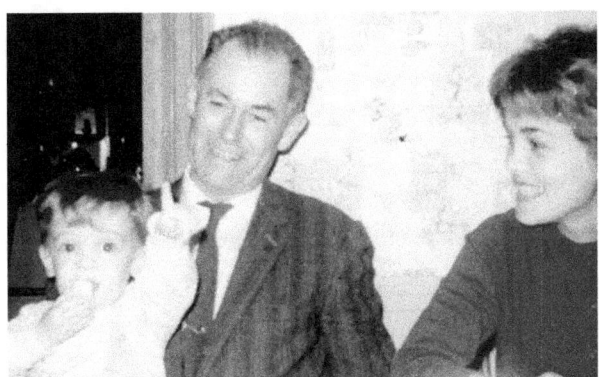

The author, apple in mouth, with his grandfather and mother way back in 1964.

CONTENTS

Author Biography   I

1 You Can Be Fit!   P. 1

2 Start Today!   P. 15

3 Aerobic Exercise   P. 29

4 Strength Training   P. 71

5 Healthy Diet Essentials   P. 121

6 Brain Boosters   P. 151

7 Special Health Conditions   P. 195

8 Fit Body Fit Mind for Life!   P. 207

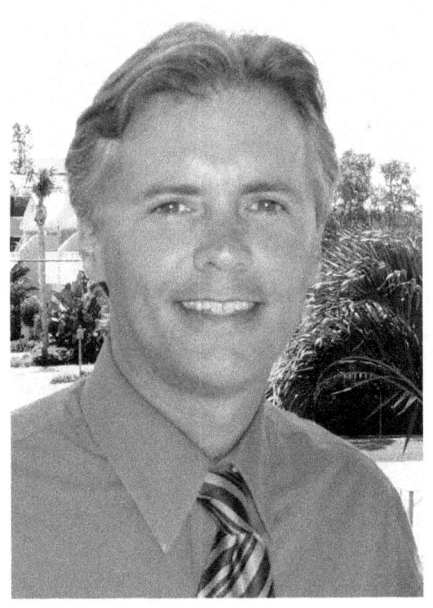

AUTHOR BIOGRAPHY

Lawrence S. Richardson, Jr., is an International Sports Sciences Association certified Senior Fitness Specialist. Richardson graduated with honors from the University of Southern California, where he double-majored in broadcast journalism and history.

A fitness enthusiast for over 30 years, Richardson drew on his experience as a journalist, columnist, and public relations, public affairs, and marketing executive to write and design this book and to create its companion website, **Xeniors.com**. Richardson is grateful to the many fitness researchers and health professionals who developed the knowledge base that made this book possible.

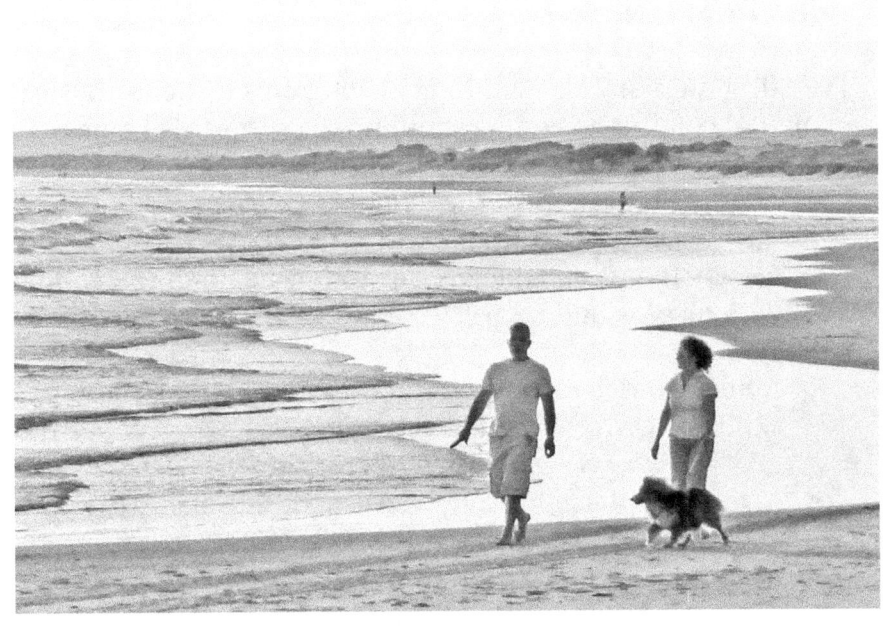

1 YOU CAN BE FIT!

Every day, millions of people just like you walk, run, cycle, swim, dance, practice yoga, lift weights, draw, paint, shoot photos, play a musical instrument, and engage in dozens of other activities that promote fit bodies and fit minds. Their dedication to an active lifestyle substantially increases the odds that they will live the long, healthy, happy, mobile, and independent lives we all desire and deserve. Here's your chance to join them!

Fit Body Fit Mind: Your Practical Guide to Aging Well was written to give you – whether an absolute beginner or experienced athlete – specific, fad-free, scientifically proven, and truly achievable techniques to improve your overall physical and mental fitness, so you, too, can get the most out of every precious day of your life. In other words, this book is for people who want to grow, not just grow old.

WHAT IS FITNESS?

The first step on the road to achieving an excellent physical and mental condition is understanding that fitness is having:

➤ A body that can meet the demands of everyday life.

➤ A body that is capable of preventing, healing, and coping with disease and injury.

➤ A body that is strong, energetic, and mobile, so you can explore new, stimulating activities.

➤ A mind that is positive, refreshed, enthusiastic, alert, and able to appreciate, absorb, and process new experiences, information, and skills.

➤ A mind that is sharp and as interested as it is interesting.

➤ A body and mind combined that allow you to interact positively with others and embrace your world.

As you can see, this list isn't just a definition of fitness, it's a set of goals for us all to work toward.

Fit Body Fit Mind: Your Practical Guide To Aging Well is one of the few books available today that provides a comprehensive, detailed, and achievable plan to improve your body and mind. It also offers advice on how to integrate fitness into your everyday life – without complicated exercises or expensive equipment – and stay motivated so you will be healthy for many years to come.

Fortunately, there are many decades' worth of credible scientific research to support the fitness recommendations in this book. *(Please visit our companion website, Xeniors.com, and enter "study" in the search window to review research that supports this book's approach.)*

In fact, health researchers have studied fitness to the point that they are beginning to repeat themselves. Not surprisingly, they are reaching the same conclusion that our parents and grandparents knew to be true:

To control your weight and have a healthy body and mind at any age, you need to combine aerobic exercise, strength training, and a healthy diet with activities that challenge your brain.

Too often this simple prescription gets lost in the haze of hyper health fads that mislead you to believe you have to, as the Superman announcer said, be "faster than a speeding bullet, more powerful than a locomotive, and able to leap tall buildings in a single bound" to be fit. The truth is, you don't, and most of the programs that take the intense, quick-fix approach ultimately injure people, which is the opposite of being fit.

In reality, all you have to do to be fit is participate in a reasonable amount of aerobic and strength training exercise with total control and proper form, eat a sensible diet comprised of real, unprocessed food, and pick up a few hobbies that interest you. The following facts regarding the benefits of adopting a healthy lifestyle speak for themselves.

FASCINATING FITNESS FACTS

If you're not convinced living a healthier lifestyle is worth the effort, consider the fact that health researchers now believe HOW we live our lives determines 70 percent of how well we will age, while genetics – the traits we inherit from our parents – influences only 30 percent. That means your fate is, for the most part, in your own hands.

If that impressive and empowering discovery isn't enough to convince you to get your body and mind in gear, consider the specific benefits that healthy living can deliver. Research proves that people who adopt a healthy lifestyle gain the power to:

> ➢ Prevent, reverse, or control certain types of cancer, cardiovascular disease, sarcopenia (age-associated muscle mass and strength loss), osteoporosis (bone tissue loss), diabetes, and weight gain.

> ➢ Reduce the risk of a heart attack by 50 percent and a stroke by 40 percent. Note: Heart disease is the leading killer of men and women over 65.

> ➢ Diminish the natural reduction in their metabolism – the rate at which bodies burn calories – that occurs with age, so they can remain fit, trim, and active. (This is especially important for women whose metabolism plummets after menopause, which can lead to weight gain.)

> ➢ Cut doctor visits to half the rate of people who are physically and mentally inactive.

> ➢ Perform with the physical and mental vitality of people many decades younger when they're in their 60s, 70s, 80s and beyond.

> ➢ Cut the risk of mental conditions, such as anxiety, dementia, and depression.

> ➢ Get more, high quality sleep.

> ➢ Maintain the strength, balance, and alertness they need to remain mobile and independent to their first century and beyond.

With all these benefits for the taking, you can see why you can't afford to sit on the sideline anymore. You need to get active and fight for your life! **Fit Body Fit Mind: Your**

Practical Guide to Aging Well will show you how with specific, step-by-step recommendations that stress the importance of challenging your body and mind in gentle, productive ways, not battling them like enemies until you're injured and fatigued.

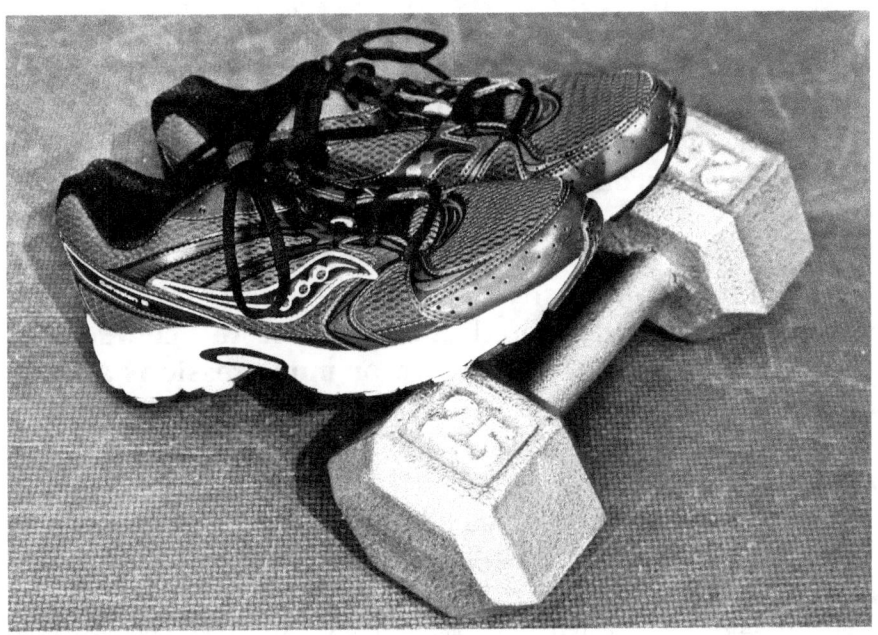

FIT BODY: 3 Essential Exercise Recommendations

The aerobic and strength training workouts and advice contained in **Fit Body Fit Mind: Your Practical Guide To Aging Well** are based on exercise recommendations established by the U.S. Health Department that are astonishingly simple, effective, and achievable. They call on generally healthy people free of serious chronic conditions or injuries to complete a reasonable amount of aerobic and strength training exercise each week.

All we need to be fit is:

1. **150 minutes of moderate-intensity aerobic exercise – such as brisk walking – each week and two or more sessions a week on non-consecutive days of muscle-strengthening activity that addresses the major muscle groups in our legs, hips, back, abdomen, chest, shoulders and arms; or**

2. **75 minutes of vigorous-intensity aerobic exercise – such as running – each week and two or more sessions a week on non-consecutive days of muscle-strengthening activity that addresses the major muscle groups; or**

3. **Any combination of moderate-intensity and vigorous-intensity aerobic exercise sessions in the time periods stated above – over the course of a week combined with two or more sessions a week on non-consecutive days of muscle-strengthening activity that addresses the major muscle groups.**

These practical recommendations are more amazingly productive than the hottest fitness fads. Imagine: All you have to do is invest about four or five of the 112 hours you're awake each week to exercise and, of course, follow a healthy diet (which we'll get to) and fitness will be yours!

The fitness recommendations are explained in detail with clearly illustrated, body-friendly, beginner and intermediate exercise routines later in this book, but following is a brief overview of each essential component.

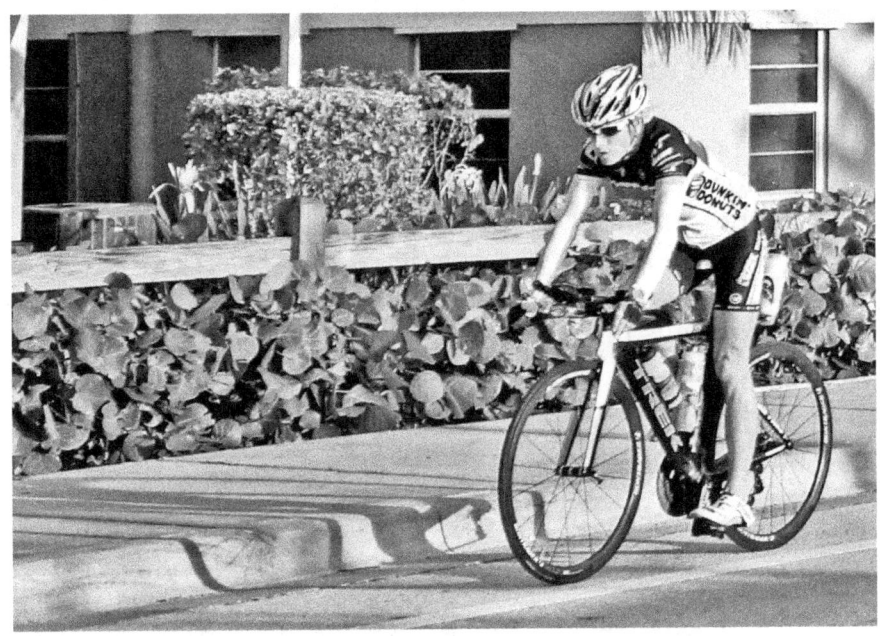

Aerobic Exercise Benefits

Aerobic exercise – walking, running, swimming, cycling, and other activities that get your heart and lungs working harder – has many health benefits. Putting your body in motion:

> ➢ Strengthens your cardiovascular system so it can more efficiently distribute oxygen and nutrients to all parts of your body while eliminating impurities.

> ➢ Reduces the risk of heart attack, stroke, obesity, diabetes, and some cancers.

> ➢ Lowers blood pressure and cholesterol levels.

> ➢ Burns calories, which is important for weight control.

> ➢ Releases endorphins – chemicals that reduce anxiety, stress and depression.

> ➢ Helps maintain and build bone density, reducing the

risk of osteoporosis. Note: Moderate impact exercises are especially good at this.

> Improves balance and mobility, which increases the odds people will be able to remain independent as they get older.

The 150 minute a week aerobic exercise time requirement seems enormous until you realize you can and should break it into smaller units. For example, walking at a brisk pace for as little as 30 minutes, five times a week or for 50 minutes, three times a week will enable you to meet the requirement.

The challenge with aerobic exercise is choosing an activity or activities that you enjoy that are appropriate for your fitness level. You want to work hard enough to collect health benefits, but not so hard that you become injured or fatigued. We'll discuss how to do this in the chapter on aerobic exercise. *(Visit Xeniors.com and enter the search term "aerobic" for relevant news and tips.)*

Aerobic exercise alone won't give you total body fitness. You also need strength training.

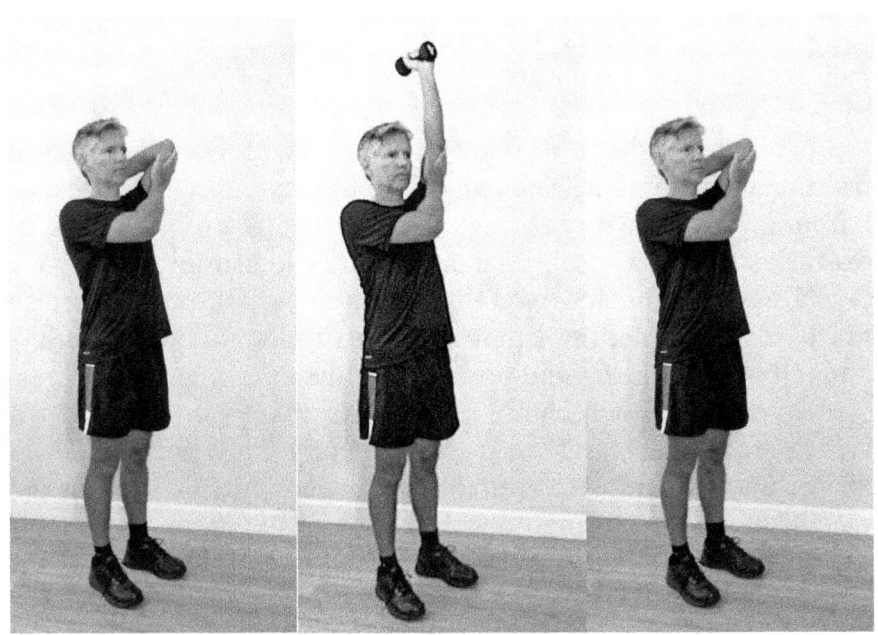

Strength Training Benefits

Strength training delivers many health benefits. Working out with resistance:

> Strengthens and maintains muscle mass, which is important to combat natural, age-related decline.

> Tones muscles, which gives them a healthy and sleek appearance.

> Reinforces and maintains the bones that make up your skeletal system, which reduces the risk of osteoporosis and fractures.

> Provides the strength, balance, and mobility needed for everyday activities while reducing the risk of falls.

> Opens the door to activities that you might not currently have the strength to participate in, such as dancing and hiking the world.

➢ Turns muscles into calorie burners, a benefit that continues even after an exercise session.

Fortunately, there are many ways to meet the strength training requirement. You can fulfill it by spending as little as a half-hour, two or three times a week completing a series of exercises that works all your major muscle groups using your own body weight, free weights, resistance bands or exercise machines. Yoga routines that work the upper and lower body – and not all do – also yield positive results.

Regardless of which form of resistance you choose, it's critical that you treat your body gently and perform each exercise with complete control and proper form. Moving the weight correctly through an entire exercise (or repetition), is the only way to ensure your body receives the greatest benefit with the least risk of injury.

Too often people try to lift too much weight and the straining, contorting, and jerking it takes to complete a repetition leads to uneven development and damage to their bodies. Sooner or later, they will suffer a catastrophic injury to their knees, hips, backs or shoulders that knocks them out of the fitness game for weeks, months or even years.

An important point to keep in mind when you participate in strength training is you and you alone are the master of your own body. If an exercise doesn't feel right – for example, you experience a sharp pain or hear joints clicking -- it's likely harming your body. To avoid injury, you need to either modify how you perform the exercise or replace it altogether with another exercise that addresses the same major muscle group.

We'll go into greater detail about how you can fulfill the strength training exercise requirement effectively, safely and enjoyably in the strength training chapter. *(Visit Xeniors.com and enter the search term "strength training" for related news and tips.)*

The last essential piece of your physical fitness program is a proper diet.

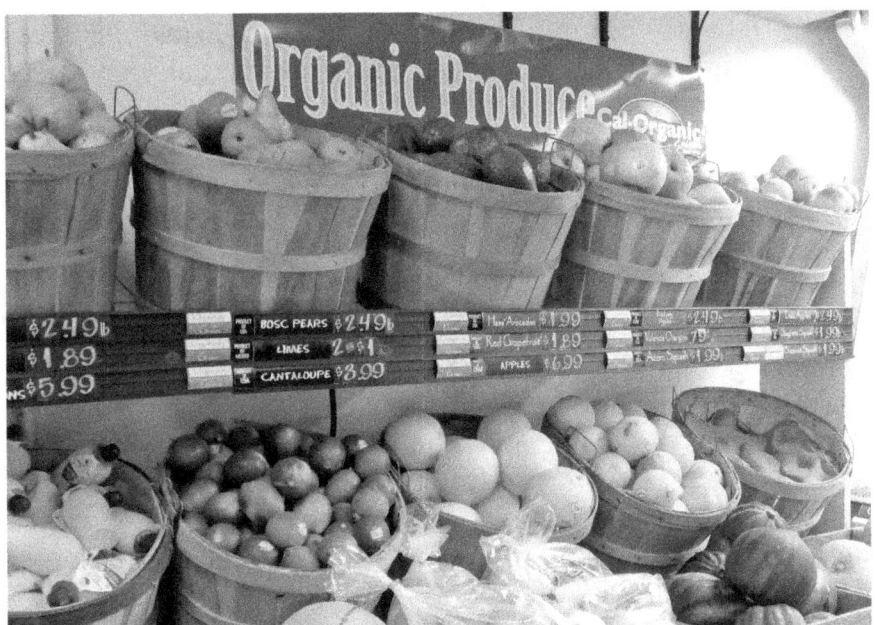

KEYS TO A HEALTHY DIET

In your quest to achieve total fitness, eating a healthy diet is every bit as important as meeting the exercise requirements. In fact, it's **more** important for people who want to lose weight.

Put simply: Food is your fuel. If you fill your body with poor quality "gas," you'll never run physically or mentally at your full potential. And, if you eat too much, you'll flood your system, and it will be harder to start.

So what is a healthy diet? A healthy diet is one that:

➢ Is rich in a variety of fresh vegetables and fruits, served raw and cooked.

➢ Substitutes whole grain rice, pastas, breads and cereals for potatoes and heavily processed grains.

➢ Restricts red meat consumption – if any at all – to a few servings a week.

➢ Delivers protein through healthy boneless, skinless white meat chicken breasts, fish, non-fat dairy products, and nuts, beans and legumes.

➢ Avoids processed foods and beverages, which are loaded with empty calories with no nutritional value and unhealthy fat, oil, sugar, and salt.

If weight loss is your major fitness goal, you should discuss a personally tailored dieting strategy with your physician or registered dietician. The group approach employed by Weight Watchers has also been shown to be more effective than going it alone.

We will describe general but effective strategies that will help most people to improve their eating habits in the chapter on dieting. There are also several healthy, vegetable rich recipes to get you started. *(Visit Xeniors.com and enter the search word "recipe" for additional meals and "diet" for the latest dieting news and tips.)*

FIT MIND: Essential Brain Boosting Activities

A healthy body provides the platform for a fit mind. Aerobic activity and strength training ensure that the brain is receiving the oxygen and nutrients it needs to thrive and fend off brain wasting diseases.

The converse is true, too. A healthy body depends on a healthy mind that is alert, refreshed and enthusiastic to get it through rigorous exercise sessions without injury. To reach this state of fitness, a mind has to be challenged by activities, such as writing a blog, reading material that forces you to think, taking up a musical instrument, painting, or photography, or volunteering in a program that requires you to learn new skills.

Researchers find that people who combine activities that challenge the mind with immersion in settings that promote positive social interaction receive many benefits, including:

> ➢ Increased blood flow to their brains, which provides the oxygen and nutrients necessary to feed a fit mind.

> ➢ More, high-quality connections between brain cells, which allows it to function quicker and more efficiently.

> ➢ Less risk of dementia as a result of the improved physical condition.

> ➢ A higher state of alertness, happiness and fulfillment than their peers who don't exercise their brains or interact with other people.

We'll discuss how to get started in several challenging but fun brain boosting activities in the chapter on mental fitness. *(Visit Xeniors.com and enter the search word "brain" for related news and tips.)*

CHRONIC HEALTH CONDITIONS

Fit Body Fit Mind: Your Practical Guide to Aging Well wouldn't be complete if it didn't discuss fitness recommendations and resources for people who are dealing with chronic health conditions, such as heart disease, high blood pressure, diabetes, arthritis, and obesity. Most people with these health challenges not only survive but thrive when they make an effort to incorporate a comprehensive fitness program into their treatment plans.

With their physician's permission and minor adaptations to exercises and activities, people of every age with chronic conditions and injuries, or those who have been sedentary their entire lives, benefit from a more active lifestyle. We'll discuss several specific approaches in the chapter on chronic conditions.

Now that you know exactly what **Fit Body Fit Mind: Your Practical Guide to Aging Well** is all about, it's time to started!

Lawrence S. Richardson, Jr.

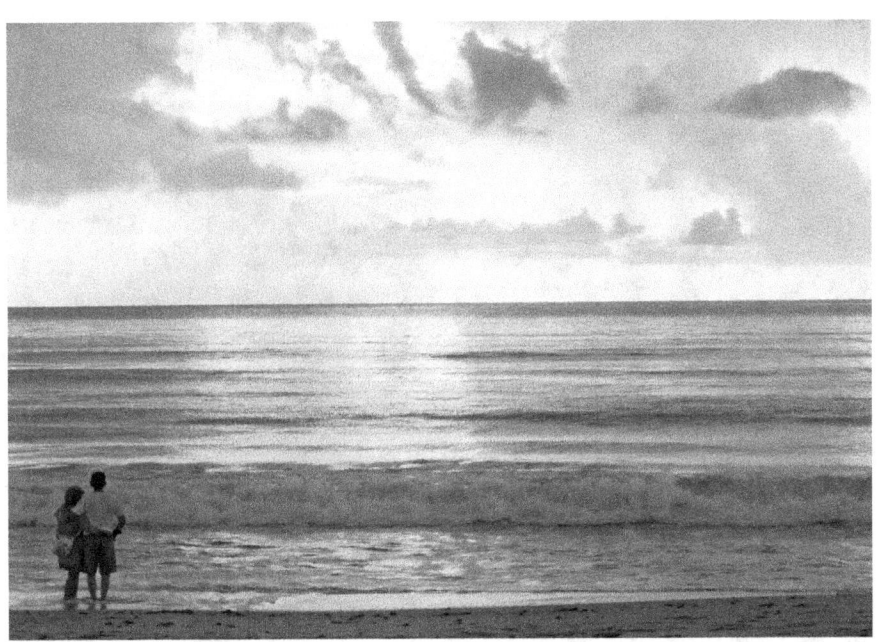

2 START TODAY!

The road to outstanding health and fitness isn't covered in a day, it's a lifetime journey, or, better yet, adventure. The first step you take toward fitness is often the most difficult. If you've been sedentary for a long time, you have to change entrenched, unhealthy habits.

One of the hardest but absolutely necessary steps is breaking the force of gravity that keeps you welded to your favorite couch or chair. Fortunately, once you get moving, you will see that being active is far more enjoyable than being inactive. Really!

Extra strength, energy, and alertness always feel better than weakness, sluggishness, and dullness of mind. Being healthy is addictive. Soon after you begin your fitness program, you'll find it increasingly easier to get up and get moving.

In addition to changing long-held unhealthy habits, you also have to change your attitude toward exercise. Instead of viewing it a special, one-time event or interruption to activities that really matter, you need to see it as a beneficial and regular part of your daily life, as important as eating, drinking and sleeping. You also absolutely have to make time for it. The following steps will help you get started.

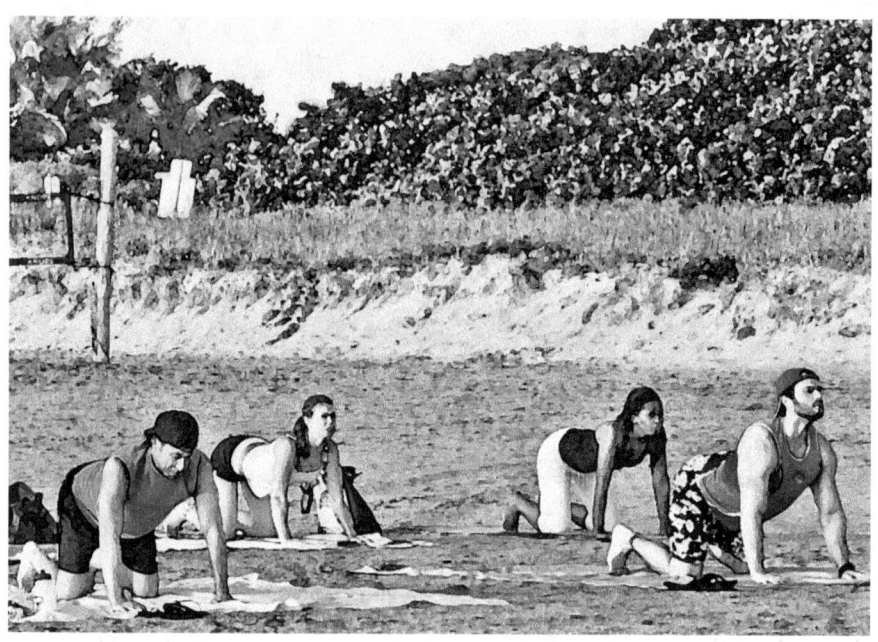

6 STEPS TO KICKSTART YOUR FITNESS PROGRAM

Getting on the road to health, fitness, and aging well will be a lot easier when you follow these six essential steps:

1. Visit Your Physician

Don't wait for tomorrow to get started on this life renewing quest. Make an appointment today to seek your doctor's permission to exercise and his or her guidance regarding activities that are appropriate for your physical condition.

When you visit your doctor, you should:

> ➢ Ask him or her to take a snapshot of your physical condition that can be used to tailor an appropriate aerobic and strength training exercise program.

➢ Discuss any pre-existing conditions that may affect your ability to exercise and strategies to treat the condition so you can exercise and/or accommodate it in your exercise program.

➢ Discuss activities that you should or should not perform based on your level of fitness and any chronic conditions or injuries.

➢ Ask for assistance choosing a form of aerobic exercise that is appropriate for your health status. For example, if you have been sedentary most of your life and are carrying extra pounds, your doctor might advise you to begin your aerobic training by walking, not running, to give your body a chance to get used to exercising and reduce the impact on your hips and knees. Or, if you have arthritis, your doctor might recommend that you participate in a non-weight-bearing exercise, like swimming, over a low-impact exercise, like walking.

➢ Ask for help choosing a form of strength training exercise that is appropriate for your physical condition. For example, if you have arthritis, hip, or knee replacements, or hypertension, heart disease, glaucoma, or other eye conditions that are sensitive to increases in blood pressure, your doctor may advise you to skip some strength training exercises that could worsen your condition.

➢ Get a referral to a registered dietician, if necessary, to discuss weight loss strategies.

You also need to ask your doctor how to tell if you're working your body at a level of intensity that yields the greatest benefits when participating in an aerobic exercise session. There are two basic methods your doctor may suggest:

Talk Test:

The simplest, but not necessarily most scientific, approach to measuring exertion during aerobic exercise is the talk test. It's based on the concept that the harder you work your heart and lungs, the more difficult it will be to carry on a conversation. Here are the basic guidelines:

> ➢ If you can talk comfortably while engaged in aerobic exercise, you're likely not working hard enough.

> ➢ If you can talk, but just barely, you're working at a good pace.

> ➢ If you're totally out of breath and can't talk at all, you're working too hard.

The talk test works fairly well for generally fit individuals, but it's not an accurate indicator of exertion for people who have pre-existing conditions, such as heart disease, lung disease, obesity or asthma, as they may more easily run out of breath.

Target Heart Rate:

Monitoring your target heart rate – based on your pulse or the number of times your heart beats per minute – is a more accurate indicator of exertion than the talk test because it takes your age into consideration. The specific equation is to take 220 and subtract your age to reach your Maximum Heart Rate. The Target Heart Rate Zone most people need to stay within for maximum health benefit is 50-85% of their Maximum Heart Rate.

> **EXAMPLE**: To calculate your Target Heart Rate at 60 years of age, you would take 220 and subtract 60, which equals a Maximum Heart Rate of 160 beats per minute. Take 160 beats per minute and multiply it by 50% and

the low end of your Target Heart Rate Zone is 80 beats per minute. Take 160 beats per minute and multiply it by 85% and the high end of your Target Heart Rate Zone is 136 beats per minute. Exercising toward the high end of your Target Heart Rate Zone will yield the greatest benefit. This is in the most general terms. **YOU MUST DISCUSS AN APPROPRIATE TARGET HEART RATE WITH YOUR PHYSICIAN.** Also be aware that some medications that affect your pulse can skew the accuracy of your target heart rate readings.

To accurately measure your heart rate (pulse), you can either use a heart rate monitor or take your pulse manually by pressing your fingertips on an artery. To take your pulse, press the pads of your index finger and middle finger – not your thumb – against the inside of your wrist or at the side of your neck just below your jaw. To calculate your pulse, count the number of beats in 15 seconds and multiply it by four or count the number of beats in 30 seconds and multiply it by two.

As you can see, your doctor is an important member of your fitness team before you begin actually exercising, but he or she also needs to play a role after you start. You need to ask your doctor to help you monitor your progress and address any pain, injury or other complicating condition that may arise during exercise.

A personal fitness trainer may also be a valuable professional to add to your fitness team.

2. Consider Hiring A Personal Fitness Trainer

Once you have your physician's permission to begin a fitness program, it's time to consider whether or not you need a certified personal fitness trainer to assist you. If you've never engaged in aerobic or strength training exercise, you want to refine your technique, or you're ready to shift your program into a higher gear with new, unfamiliar exercises, hiring a personal fitness trainer is a smart move.

As your personal coach, a fitness trainer can:

➢ Conduct tests to objectively evaluate your level of fitness.

➢ Design an effective aerobic and strength training exercise program – by conferring with your physician and/or physical therapist, when necessary – that accommodates your fitness level and any pre-existing conditions.

➢ Help you to choose a variety of aerobic and strength training exercises that will enable you to meet your fitness goals.

➢ Show you how to exercise with total control and proper form to get the most out of each repetition and avoid injury.

➢ Modify or replace exercises that are causing pain or injury.

➢ Track your progress and adjust your routine whenever necessary to yield better results.

➢ Address any unusual conditions that may arise during or after your exercise session.

➢ Monitor your health if you have a chronic condition that's sensitive to exertion, such as heart disease, high blood pressure, or diabetes.

➢ Motivate you to continue exercising.

You are going to spend a lot of time with your personal trainer, so make sure you find one who is a good fit. Your personal trainer should:

➢ Have the education necessary to address your specific goals, challenges and conditions.

➢ Have a personality that complements yours.

➢ Be positive, supportive and encouraging.

➢ Pay sole attention to you when you're exercising.

➢ Provide constant guidance on the proper way to execute an exercise so you will get the greatest benefit and avoid injury.

➢ Challenge you in ways that promote your health and well-being, instead of pushing you to work harder than is safe for your body.

➢ Address any injuries in a responsible manner by not making you power through the pain.

➢ Refer you to your doctor or another specialist when you have a question he or she is not qualified to answer.

➢ Give you regular reports on where you're making progress and where you need to work harder.

When working with a personal fitness trainer, it's important to remember you are working as a team. Only do what feels right and productive for your body and don't be afraid to question your trainer about exercises that seem counter-productive. A good trainer will welcome your feedback and gladly alter your fitness program.

3. Team Up With A Buddy

Exercising with a buddy is a great way to keep your workout sessions fun and to stay motivated. Realize, however, when you're searching for a workout buddy that you can't make someone else exercise. If your partner, spouse or friend isn't really into fitness, find someone who is. The last thing you need is a buddy who's a downer.

The qualities you should seek in an exercise buddy are the same qualities you should expect from yourself. He or she should be:

> ➤ Truly interested in improving their fitness level.

> ➤ Dedicated to showing up on time and prepared to exercise.

> ➤ As enthusiastic as you are about exercise, which will build a positive synergy that will keep you both motivated.

> ➤ Of similar physical ability so you're not holding each other back. (If you're not quite a perfect match, you can exercise with your buddy part of the time then make up the difference on your own.)

> ➤ Willing to learn proper form so you can prompt each other when needed.

One important note: If your buddy drops out, do not use their failure as an excuse to quit, too. You are responsible for your own health and well-being.

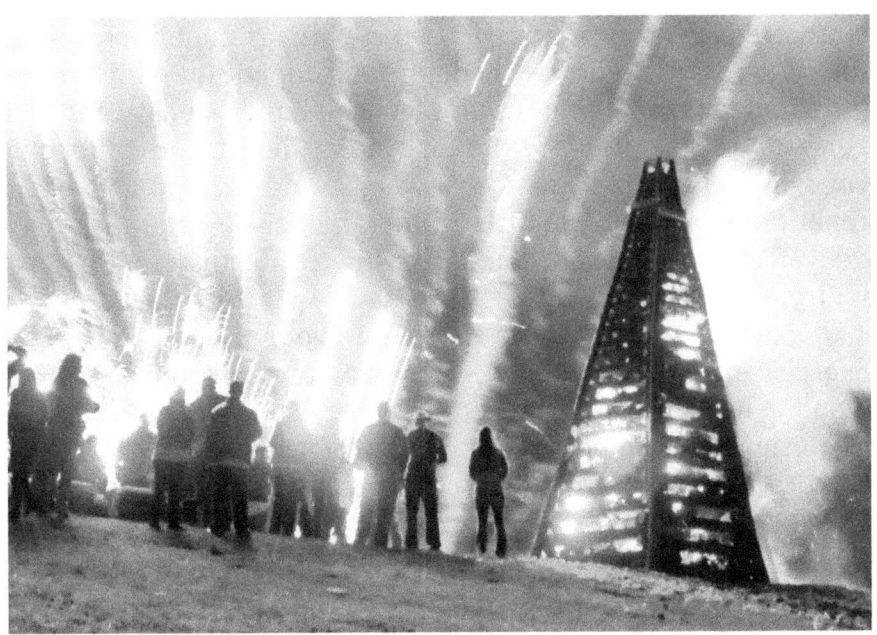

4. Fight Flame-out

We all know people who buy a new treadmill, stationary bike, or other piece of exercise equipment and enthusiastically commit to using it for two hours every night. (Maybe we've even done it ourselves.) They usually last about a week or two before they're bored or injured or both and give up. Don't be one of them!

Take the responsible approach and remember you don't need to commit two hours a day to exercising when as little as thirty minutes a day will yield positive results. Taking a mature and measured approach will always win over the overly-enthusiastic and unrealistic approach.

If you have been inactive for a long time, you need to phase in your exercise program very gradually. The government's recommended number of minutes you should devote to working out each week is for people who are active and have built up the ability to go for longer periods of time.

When you begin your aerobic exercise program, start with short walks, as little as five or ten minutes, and slowly add additional minutes as you become more fit. When you begin your strength training program, start with an amount of weight that you can easily move through each repetition with proper form and control for eight times. As you build strength and can perform 12 repetitions without straining, jerking or contorting your body, add a little more weight and go back to eight repetitions again. This slow and deliberate approach will deliver the most health benefits while protecting you against injury.

It's also important to be realistic in your expectations. Fad exercise programs and fad diets that promise quick results won't deliver fitness for a lifetime. They'll only serve to set you up for injury, disappointment and burnout. Take the slow, safe road to fitness, and you will reap health benefits for years to come.

5. Stay Motivated

Studies show that most people who take up a fitness program quit exercising within a month. This is usually because they start out with unrealistic expectations of what their bodies can accomplish – weight loss chief among them – in a short period of time. You don't have to be one of them.

To improve the odds that you will stay in the fitness game:

➤ Focus on realistic, achievable, long-term goals that will ensure you build a healthy body, not destructive short term goals.

➤ Choose sports and activities that you truly enjoy.

➤ Join a gym, club, or class with others who share your interests.

➤ Try a new gym or change your aerobic exercise route to breathe life into your workouts.

➤ Hire a personal trainer to cheer you on and provide new exercises and activities you never considered.

➤ Exercise with a buddy who makes you want to work out.

➤ Socialize with people who are positive and supportive of your fitness efforts and ignore the naysayers who want to hold you back.

➤ Shake up your exercise routine. If you're a runner or a walker, consider swimming, biking or dancing every now and then. When strength training, remember there are several exercises to work each major muscle group. Swap them out from time to time to keep things interesting. Changing the order and pacing of your exercise routine can also create new and interesting challenges.

➤ Challenge yourself by entering condition-appropriate road races and competitions.

➤ Play this mind game: On the days you least want to exercise – when it's not due to illness or injury – force yourself to get up and go. You'll be surprised at how much better you will feel after you exercise!

➤ Reward yourself for reaching fitness milestones or for just hanging in there with healthy prizes, like new exercise clothing and gear, dinner out, or a trip.

Keeping yourself motivated is critically important to your ability to achieve fitness for a lifetime. Try and think of rewards that will keep you in the game beyond the list that appears above.

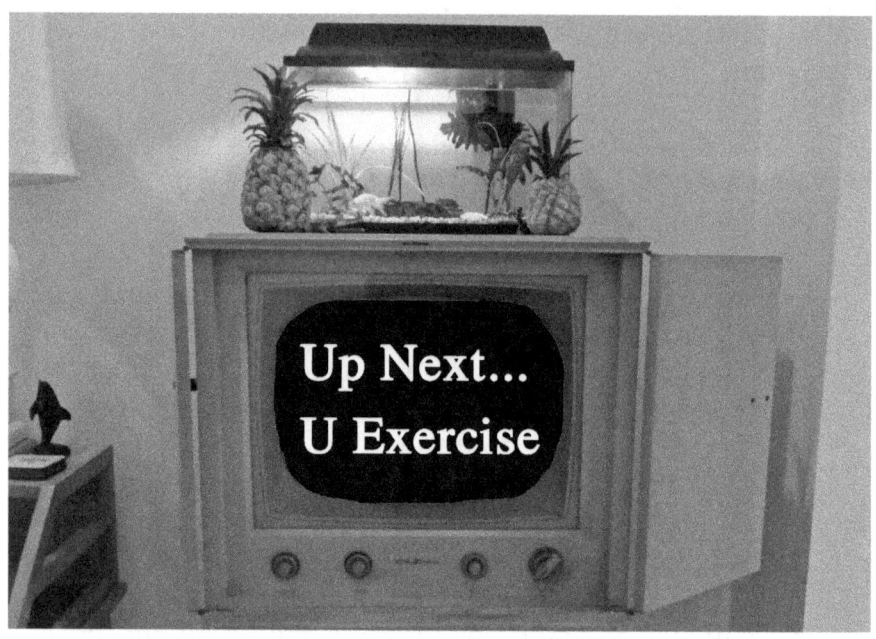

6. Take The Xeniors.com TV Challenge!

Our companion website, **Xeniors.com**, is dedicated to sharing the latest information to help you become more fit and age well. A key part of that advice is the **Xeniors.com TV Challenge**.

The challenge is simple: Many of us spend the equivalent of a day or more each week watching television. At least once a day, a show comes on that we don't really like or we've seen a hundred times before, but, for want of anything else to do, we watch it anyway.

The Xeniors.com TV Challenge calls on all of us to use that one show as a cue to get up and exercise. Spend five half-hour shows or three one-hour shows a week taking a brisk walk and your fitness level will improve. Spend two or three half-hour shows a week strength training and you'll be amazed at the results.

Please visit Xeniors.com and let us know if the TV Challenge works for you. Your stories will help others to get involved.

YOU CAN DO IT!

Every day, health researchers release studies in support of aerobic exercise, strength training, a healthy diet, and activities that develop an active mind as the four pillars necessary to support whole body and mind fitness and aging well. Now it's time for you to act on their recommendations!

Follow the sensible, detailed steps in **Fit Body Fit Mind: Your Practical Guide to Aging Well** and you will be well on your way to a lifetime of good health. You will feel better physically and mentally, and your new found zest for life will have a profound, positive affect on you and the world around you.

Don't wait for tomorrow to get started on this quest. Make an appointment today to get your physician's permission to exercise, then get started!

The following chapters will give all the detailed information you need to begin your aerobic and strength training exercise programs and to challenge your mind. Enjoy!

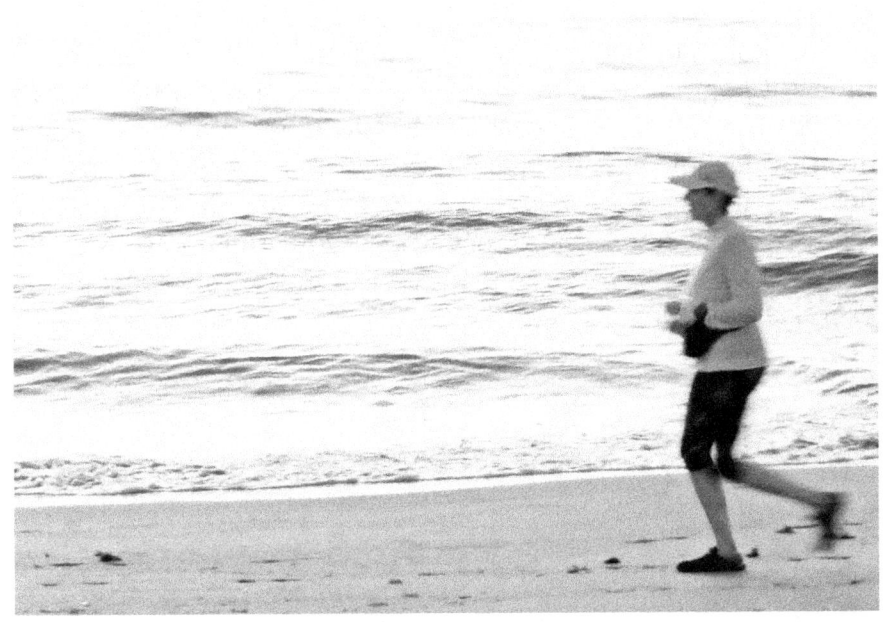

3 AEROBIC EXERCISE

Aerobic Exercise Requirement:

➢ **150 minutes of moderate-intensity aerobic exercise a week – such as brisk walking; or**

➢ **75 minutes of vigorous-intensity aerobic exercise a week – such as jogging or running ; or**

➢ **Any combination of moderate-intensity and vigorous-intensity aerobic activity in the time periods stated above over the course of a week.**

Aerobic exercise has an enormous positive impact on our bodies and minds. To walk, run, swim, ride a bike, dance, or participate in any other activity that gets our lungs heaving and our hearts pumping faster, delivers life-sustaining oxygen and nutrients to every part of our body and a natural high like no other.

As stated in the last chapter, the first thing you need to do BEFORE beginning an aerobic training program is **GET YOUR PHYSICIAN'S PERMISSION TO EXERCISE!** While extremely healthy, aerobic exercise also increases the stress load on your body, including your heart, circulatory system, lungs, muscles, joints, tendons, and bones. You need your doctor to evaluate your physical condition and to advise you on an appropriate exercise regimen.

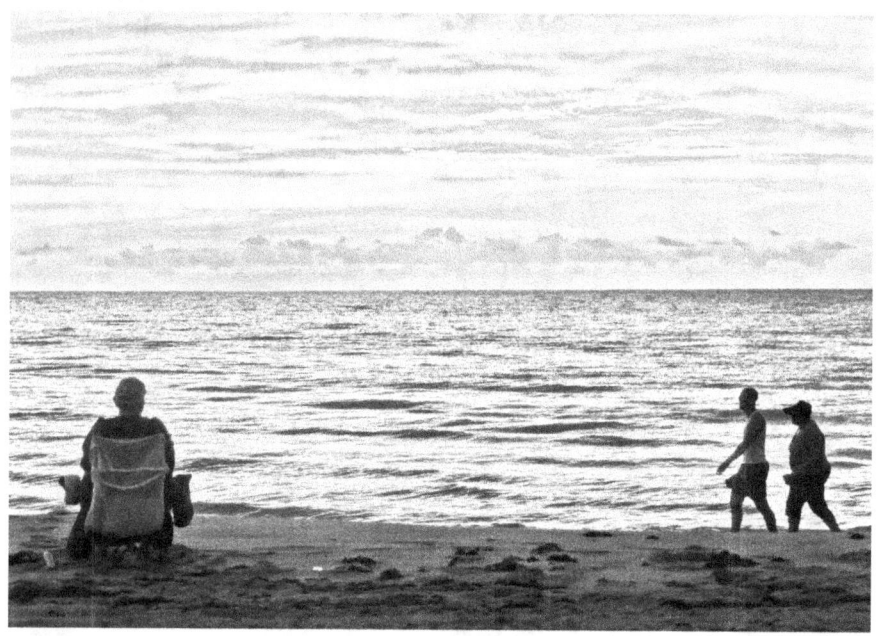

CHOOSE YOUR AEROBIC EXERCISE

Once you get your physician's permission to exercise, use his or her advice to choose your aerobic activity. Each activity has pluses and minuses that need to be considered. For example:

➢ Walking briskly is a great, low-impact aerobic exercise that delivers maximum benefits but it can require a substantial investment in time.

➢ Running, on the other hand, delivers the same health benefits as a brisk walk in about half the time, but it is higher impact, which can be tough on ankles, knees and hips.

➢ Swimming laps is good for your cardiovascular system and strengthens your arms and shoulders. As a non-load bearing exercise, it's superb for people with musculoskeletal issues such as arthritis. However, it does not build muscle throughout your body or protect bones from osteoporosis. (This deficit can be made up during your strength training sessions, which are discussed in detail in the next chapter.)

➢ Dancing, especially with a partner, can be low-impact or high-impact, depending on the style of dance. It also has a strength training component as you lead or follow your partner across the floor. Finding opportunities to dance on a regular basis, however, can be a challenge.

In addition to knowing the strengths and weaknesses of each aerobic activity when making your choice, it's also important to consider whether or not you actually like an activity. If you like it, you will stay with it. If you don't, you're at risk of quitting. Another way to stay in the fitness game is by participating in a variety of activities each week. The varied experiences will help you to remain interested and enthusiastic.

Another point to consider is where you prefer to exercise. Indoor aerobic exercise performed at home or in a gym is excellent for people who don't like to deal with weather extremes, pollution and allergens, or potential hazards found on outdoor courses. They can exercise on machines – such as treadmills, elliptical trainers, stationary bikes – or in swimming pools. They can also take step aerobics or dance classes. There are also many excellent aerobic exercise DVDs that they can use at home during their workout sessions.

Machines, such as treadmills and stationary bikes, are great because most allow you to adjust the speed, length or difficulty of your workout. They also have electronic systems to measure time, pace, distance, heart rate and calories expended. Just make sure whatever machine you choose is properly adjusted for your body size, and that it does not put undue stress on your ankles, knees or hips.

Group classes, such as step aerobics and dance, provide the dual benefits of high quality aerobic exercise and the opportunity to socialize, which helps participants to stay motivated. Exercise in the low to moderate impact range is best for your body. High impact exercise puts you at risk of injuring your lower body.

Once you choose your aerobic exercise, you need to purchase activity-appropriate clothing and gear.

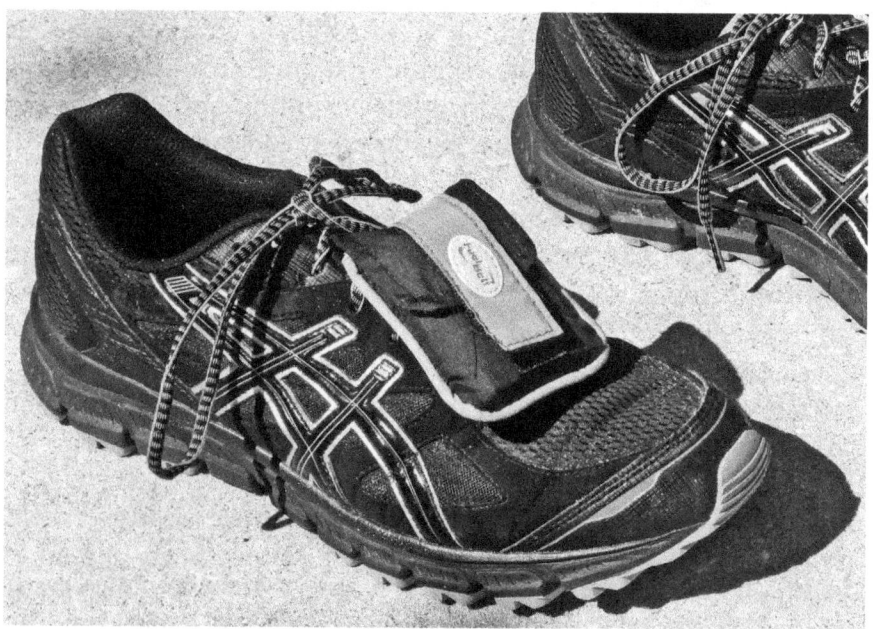

BUY THE RIGHT GEAR

The most important point to keep in mind when purchasing exercise clothing and gear is: COMFORT COUNTS! Clothing and sports equipment is supposed to serve you. That means you shouldn't have to bear discomfort or adapt in any way to accommodate it. *(Enter the keyword "gear" into the search field on Xeniors.com or click on the "Great Gear & Gifts" button on the top of the homepage for gear reviews and recommendations.)*

Sports Shoes

Aerobic exercise clothing begins at your feet. You need to find sports shoes that are so comfortable you don't realize they're there. Look for shoes that:

> ➢ Are light weight.

> ➢ Fit comfortably from toe to arch to heel.

> ➢ Are made of mesh material that breathes and doesn't abrade your feet.

> ➢ Feature an upper structure that includes reinforcing bands connected to the soles to hold your feet firmly in place. Some fad shoes are being marketed without such reinforcement, which allows your feet to shift around.

> ➢ Have heel cups that hold your heels in place but don't abrade your ankles or Achilles' tendons.

> ➢ Have simple soles, not odd space-age innovations, like bubbler shock absorbers, springs or wavy treads – all of which will serve to throw your feet off center when they impact the ground, which can damage your ankles, knees and hips.

If you purchase sports shoes that don't feel right, take them back to the store. Shoes that fall short of your expectations won't miraculously change with frequent use. They will at best annoy you and at worst cause injury – both of which put you at greater risk for dropping out before you even get started.

Clothing

Sports clothing, too, must meet these high standards. You need to buy athletic socks, undergarments, shorts, shirts, sweatpants, and sweat jackets that are:

> ➤ Season-appropriate so you do not become too cold in winter or overheat in summer.

> ➤ Made primarily of synthetic materials that, unlike cotton or wool, wick perspiration away from your body without becoming hot, soggy or heavy.

> ➤ Loose enough to allow you to breathe, yet not so loose they get in your way.

> ➤ Easy to wear in layers that can be added or removed if you become too cold or hot.

> ➤ Free of manufacturing defects that abrade your skin or cause you to lose correct form.

> ➤ Designed with light or bright colors that can easily be seen by drivers when you're exercising outdoors.

The point here is that you want sports clothing that performs at such a high standard you don't know it's there. That way, instead of constantly adjusting your clothes, you can spend all your time enjoying your aerobic workout.

Sports shoes and clothing are subject to wear and tear. When they inevitably become uncomfortable, replace them. Walking and running shoes with unevenly worn treads can cause misalignment of ankles, knees and hips that can result in injury. Don't be surprised if you have to buy new ones every six months.

Sports Gear

In addition to basic clothing, you should also consider purchasing the following gear to make your aerobic exercise sessions more enjoyable, especially if you're exercising outdoors:

➢ A light weight, brimmed cap to block the sun and prevent sweat from dripping into your eyes.

➢ Wrap-around sports sunglasses with SPF-rated lenses that can prevent the sun's dangerous ultra-violet rays from damaging your eyes.

➢ A sunglasses retainer cord to keep your sunglasses from slipping off your face.

➢ A bandanna you can tie around your wrist and use to wipe excess sweat from your brow.

➢ A GPS watch with heart rate monitor to keep track of your time, distance, and pace on the road and ensure you reach your target heart rate.

➢ Zinc oxide sunblock to protect your nose, ears, and face from the sun's harmful rays.

➢ A broad spectrum, sports sunscreen and lip balm with an SPF rating of 15 or higher to prevent the rest of your exposed skin from burning.

➢ A shoe safe, a small pocket that attaches to your laces, that can hold your keys, ID, health insurance card and cash. (Never hide your keys under a welcome mat or potted plant, where observant thieves can retrieve them.)

One final purchase to consider is a personal music player.

Many people find music enjoyable while they're exercising. Up-tempo music can also actually inspire us to work harder.

Today's music players, which play MP3s or Apple's iTunes format, come in sizes so small they can be clipped onto clothing. My favorite music player is a headset sold by Sony that doesn't have earphone cords that can tangle in your limbs or thump inside your ears when you're in motion. *(Enter "Walkman" in the search window on Xeniors.com to read a review about the player.)*

If you do decide to use a music player, make sure to keep the volume down low enough to prevent damaging your ears and so you can clearly hear the world around you. Also, be careful not to become so distracted switching tracks that you run into people, poles, or out into the street.

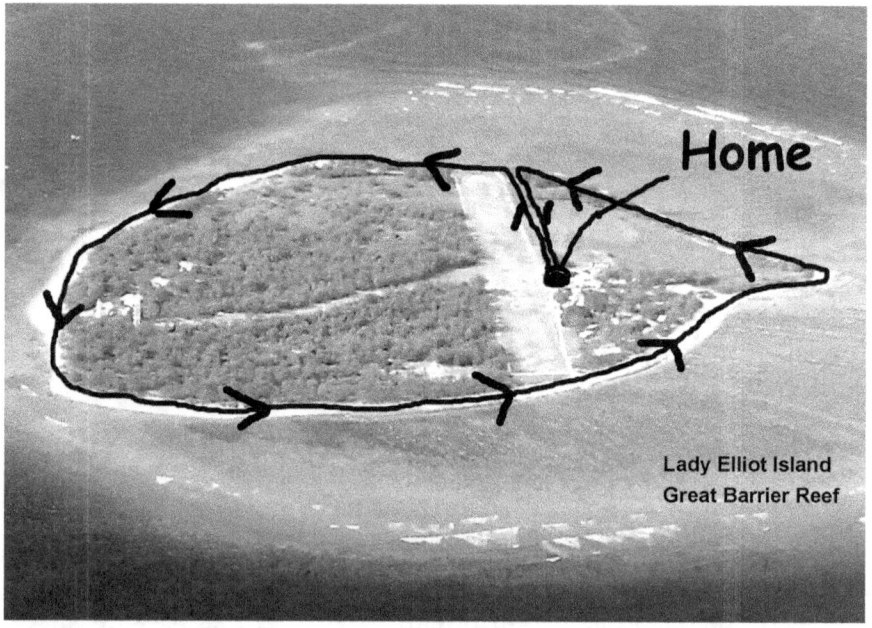

Home

**Lady Elliot Island
Great Barrier Reef**

MAP A ROUTE

If you're exercising outdoors, you should choose a route that:

> ➤ Has sidewalks and is well lit to keep you safe from

traffic.

➤ Is well-travelled by others, especially if you exercise alone.

➤ Is free of dangerous animals (the most common being dogs).

➤ Has an even, well-maintained surface free of obstructions or holes that may cause you to trip.

➤ Is level or has hills that you can handle at your fitness level.

➤ Never travels so far from your home that getting back is a problem. Using your home as a center point with the route traveling a radius around it is a good idea.

➤ Has water fountains, bathrooms, and other facilities you may need along the way. Public parks with facilities make excellent mid-points.

➤ Includes natural beauty or points of interest that keep you inspired.

Even if you find the perfect route, don't ever assume drivers can see you. Cell phone talkers and texters are increasingly running into other cars, cyclists and pedestrians, which means you have to be alert to drivers at all times and only cross the street when you're sure they see you.

After you map out your route, drive it to make sure it's safe and appropriate for your fitness level. Also, let someone know your route so they can find you if you're overdue. For added protection, wear a shoe safe that contains your identification, emergency contact number, insurance information and money, in case you need to buy water or food or make a call.

10 FREQUENTLY ASKED QUESTIONS

1. **What time should I exercise?** You should exercise at whatever time is comfortable for you. Some people are at their best first thing in the morning, while others prefer early evening. Nighttime exercise is not generally recommended because it may hinder your sleep. In summer, you can avoid the sun's intense rays and heat of day by exercising in the early morning or late afternoon. In winter, you might want to exercise in daylight hours when you will be more visible to drivers.

2. **Should I eat or drink before I exercise?** Eating and being well-hydrated is a good idea before you exercise, but being too full isn't. Try to eat and drink at least an hour before you engage in aerobic exercise.

3. **How long should I exercise?** If you're not fit, you should gradually phase in exercise. Start with five to ten minutes per session and then add minutes as you become fitter. When you reach your maximum intended length of time – usually 45 minutes to an hour per session – you can pick up your pace or add some hills to challenge your body.

4. **Should I exercise for time or distance?** Beginners should ignore time and distance and take on only as much exercise as they can handle with proper form. As you become more fit, you can exercise for a set period of time. Be careful, however, that you don't try to cover a set distance in a set amount of time before you're ready or you may find yourself sacrificing safety and proper form in a struggle to reach the finish line.

5. **Should I exercise through pain?** In a word: No. Exerting yourself and maybe even experiencing sore muscles, especially when you're just beginning or when you increase your time or distance, is normal.

Experiencing cramps, pulls, or tearing in muscles, tightening in tendons, or pain in major internal organs, such as your heart, lungs, or stomach, is not. When this happens, you need to stop, evaluate the source of the problem, and determine whether you can modify your workout and continue without injury. If not, go home and research how to deal with the pain before your next workout. **If your pain is serious, immediately call for medical assistance or see your physician.**

6. **Should I exercise when I'm ill or injured.** No, again. Illness or injury is your body's way of telling you it needs to rest so it can heal. Exercising when you're ill or injured puts you at risk of developing serious complications that will inevitably prevent you from exercising for a lot longer than if you had given your body the break it needed. Rest, recover, and regain your strength before you return to your regular workouts. And don't feel guilty about the time off. There are 365 days in a year and even a few lost weeks aren't reason to despair.

7. **What should I do if I experience the symptoms of heat exhaustion or heat stroke?** The symptoms of heat exhaustion and its more serious advanced version heat stroke include: Exhaustion, fatigue, muscle cramping, chills, dizziness, headaches, excessive sweating, nausea, vomiting, confusion, dry skin, rapid heartbeat, shortness of breath, confusion, loss of consciousness, and convulsions. There's a fine line between heat exhaustion and heat stroke, and the symptoms can come on fast in hot, humid weather. If you experience the early symptoms, stop what you're doing, seek a cool shady area, and drink plenty of water. **If the symptoms persist or worsen, seek medical assistance as heat stroke can result in death.**

8. **Should I exercise alone?** Ideally, you should exercise

with a buddy in case you experience distress. If that's not possible, exercise in an area – like a mall, a gym, or a public park – where other people can help you if necessary.

9. **Should I exercise in inclement weather?** Walking or running outdoors on a warm, showery day shouldn't be a problem. Exercising outdoors on extreme weather days – during snowstorms, ice storms, thunderstorms, heavy, blinding rain, or when heat advisories are posted – is not recommended. On those days, exercise indoors using aerobic exercise machines – such as a treadmill, stationary bike or elliptical machine – or to an aerobic exercise DVD. *(Visit Xeniors.com and enter the search word "DVD" to see our buying guide.)*

10. **What should I do if I'm injured?** Stop what you're doing and evaluate the severity of the injury. If it's serious – a broken bone or torn hamstring or Achilles' tendon – seek immediate medical attention. If it's minor – an ankle sprain or shin splints – try treating it by applying ice wrapped in a face cloth to the affected area for no more than twenty minutes at a time for up to 48 hours after the initial injury. After that, you may need to apply warm to hot towels to the injury to promote blood flow and loosen and relax the injured area. Do not resume your regular exercise activities until the injured area has fully recovered. Exercising before then puts you at risk of re-injuring the damaged area or causing you to exercise with improper form, which can have a negative impact on the rest of your body. Also, be careful not to use elbow, knee, or back supports without your doctor's permission, as they can result in muscle atrophy.

LET'S EXERCISE!

WARM UP

Now that you're all suited up and ready to go, it's important to spend five to ten minutes warming up your body. Your muscles need to be warmed up to extend and contract without cramping or tearing.

Before aerobic exercise, you should walk for five to ten minutes at your regular, not accelerated, walking pace until you just begin to break a sweat. On cold winter days, jogging in place indoors will help you to warm up before you head outdoors.

Stretching, much to most people's surprise, is not recommended before exercise. Research indicates that too much stretching actually puts your body at greater risk of injury by loosening muscles and tendons to the point that they can't keep your musculoskeletal system in proper alignment during an exercise session.

That said, if you have a specific problem area, such as tight Achilles' tendons, calves, or hamstrings, a little gentle stretching is a good idea. Just don't overdo it.

EXERCISE

Once you're warmed up, it's time to exercise. Each aerobic exercise has specific requirements for proper form. Following are tips for the most popular activities, walking and running. We'll feature tips for other activities, like swimming, cycling, and dancing, at the end of this chapter.

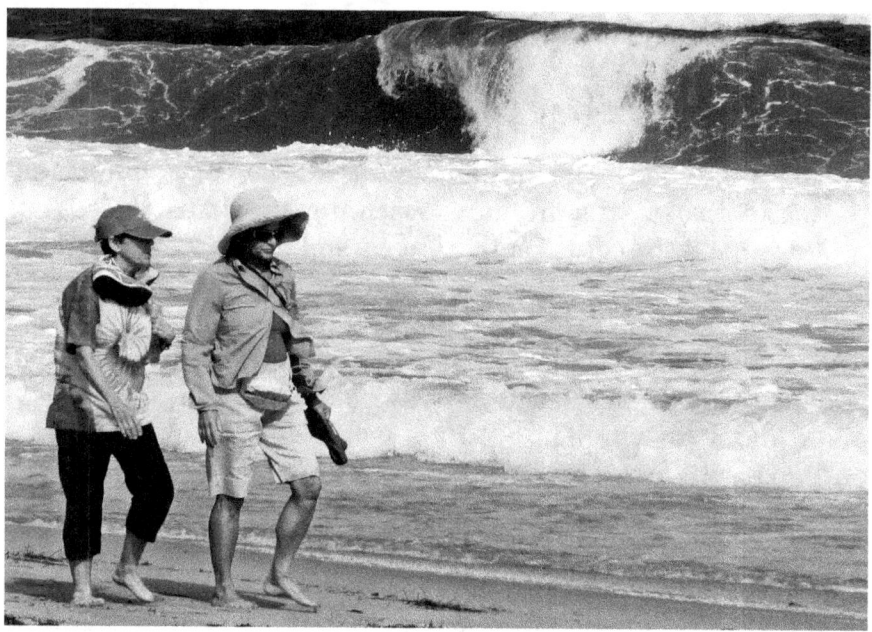

Walking

When you're walking, the proper form is to:

➢ Look forward but with a slight downward tilt to your head so you can see obstructions on the surface in front of you.

➢ Have your head, neck, and back in a straight line and your shoulders and hips facing forward and parallel to the ground.

➢ Your arms should swing by your sides with a slight bend at the elbows.

➢ Maintain control over your body by engaging your core – abdomen and back muscles – but be careful not to tense up your hands, arms, neck and shoulders. Tension is a waste of energy that can lead to unnecessary soreness.

> ➢ Your feet should roll from heel to toe and never clomp on the ground. If you're clomping, you may need a different pair of shoes.

> ➢ Relax and breathe deeply. Deep breaths are more effective at oxygenating your body than short, "sippy" breaths created by forcing your rib cage to move in and out. A sure sign you're breathing correctly is feeling your abdomen inflating and deflating.

> ➢ If you begin to lose correct posture and start hunching shoulders, stooping forward, or losing an even gait, you're fatigued and need to stop exercising to avoid injury.

These tips should help you to enjoy the easiest, most natural and enjoyable exercise of all.

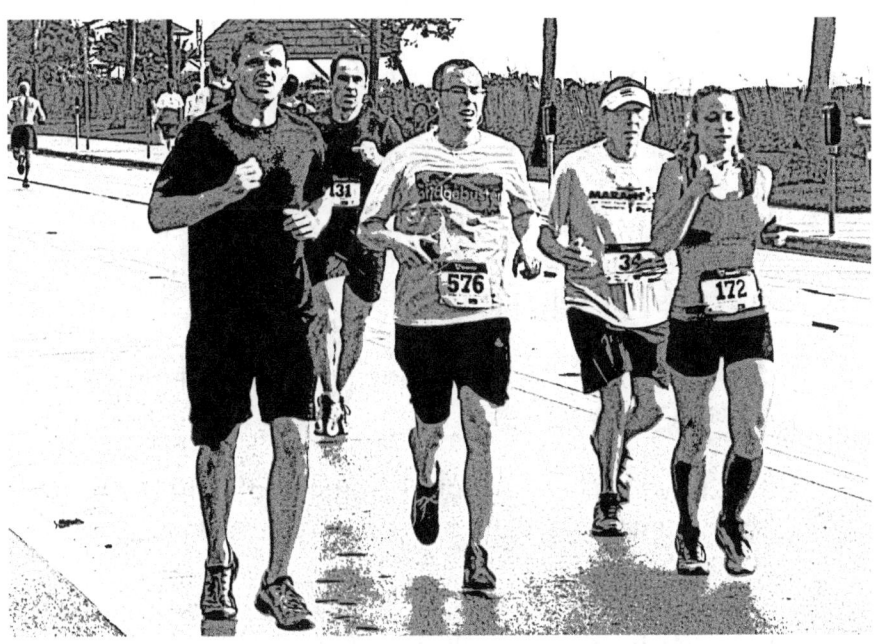

Running

Running uses the same general principles as walking with

the following minor changes to achieve proper form. When you're running, you need:

> A straight, upright posture with your shoulders and hips facing forward and parallel to the ground.

> Arms positioned at close to a 90 degree angle at the elbows and swinging by your sides with your hands traveling from your waist to close to your lower rib cage. (Some runners find it more comfortable and relaxing to keep their hands low enough that their wrists pass their outer hips.)

> Knees lifting higher than when you're walking but not too high.

> Lower legs striding further than when you walk, but not too far in front of your body.

Running is a high impact aerobic sport that requires attention to detail to avoid injury. Common running mistakes include:

> Holding your arms inward across the chest, which builds tension in your neck, shoulders, and arms and prevents full, relaxed breathing.

> Not swinging your arms enough to offset the pendulum force of your legs.

> Putting tension in your shoulders and holding them high when they should be completely relaxed.

> Trying to build speed by extending your lower leg too far forward when quicker, regular strides are more effective.

> Becoming fatigued and hunching forward or losing

shoulder alignment, which throws off your whole body.

> Making tight fists, which builds tension throughout your body, instead of allowing your hands to relax.

> Breaking proper form to hold a music player.

Run with correct posture and avoid these common mistakes and you'll find the exercise much more enjoyable and productive.

COOL DOWN AND STRETCHING

After an aerobic exercise session, it's important to cool down and stretch. The cool down should consist of five to ten minutes of walking at your regular pace, which will give your body time to recover by filtering out impurities and slowing your heart rate.

After your cool down, you should engage in 10-15 minutes of gentle stretching. Stretching prevents your muscles from tensing up, improves flexibility and blood flow, and decreases the risk of injury. Stretching can also promote a state of calmness very similar to that experienced by yoga practitioners.

The key points to keep in mind when stretching is that it must be performed with proper form to deliver maximum health benefits and minimize the risk of injury. It's also all about relaxation. When you stretch, be gentle with your body. Don't contort your body, bounce on the muscle being stretched, or use force to stretch it beyond its normal range of motion.

IMPORTANT: If you have health issues – such as heart disease, high blood pressure, eye problems, arthritis, hip or knee implants, or trouble balancing – consult with your physician to see which stretching exercises are safe for you to perform. In many instances, your doctor will advise you to avoid stretches that require you to bend forward, which can exacerbate your condition.

Stretching Routine

Following are beginner and intermediate stretching routines. Each version touches on all the major muscle groups and takes 10-15 minutes to complete. *(Visit Xeniors.com and enter the search word "stretching" to view videos that demonstrate these stretches.)*

BEGINNER STRETCHES

These stretches are for people just starting on the road to fitness or for those who have health, mobility, or balancing issues. Perform each of these stretches three times and hold them for 15-30 seconds. **If you have had neck, back, hip, or knee surgery, absolutely get your physician's permission before stretching or exercising.**

Lying Stretches

Lying stretches are good for people who have trouble balancing while standing but who have no trouble getting down and up off the floor. If you can't perform floor exercises, move directly to stretching panel #3 which address the same muscles.

1. Back of the Leg Stretch

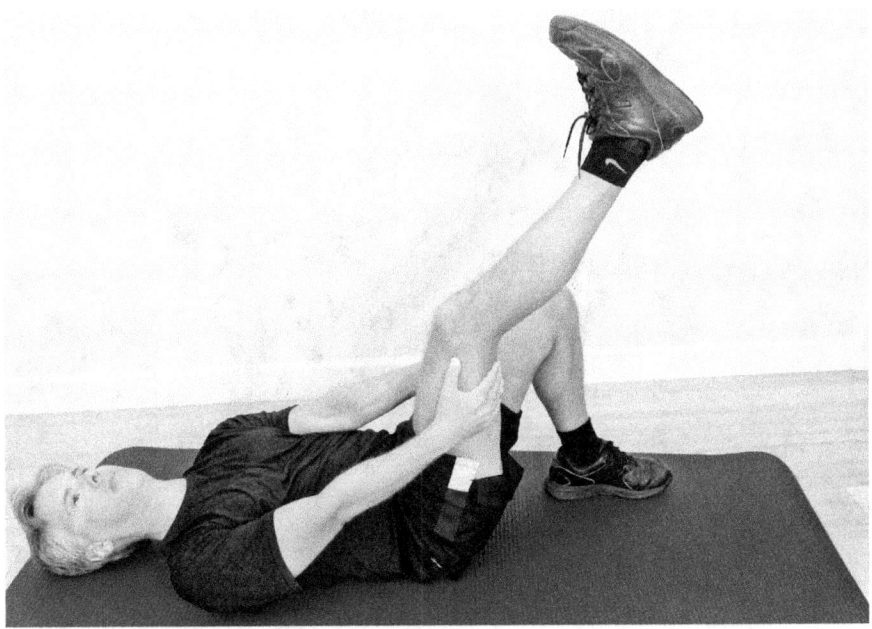

Lie on your back and bend your knees. With your head and shoulders on the mat, grasp the back of your thigh or calf. With knee slightly bent, extend your lower leg and gently pull back on your leg. You should feel the stretch in the back of your thigh. Hold for 15-30 seconds and repeat 3 times for each leg.

2. Thigh Stretch

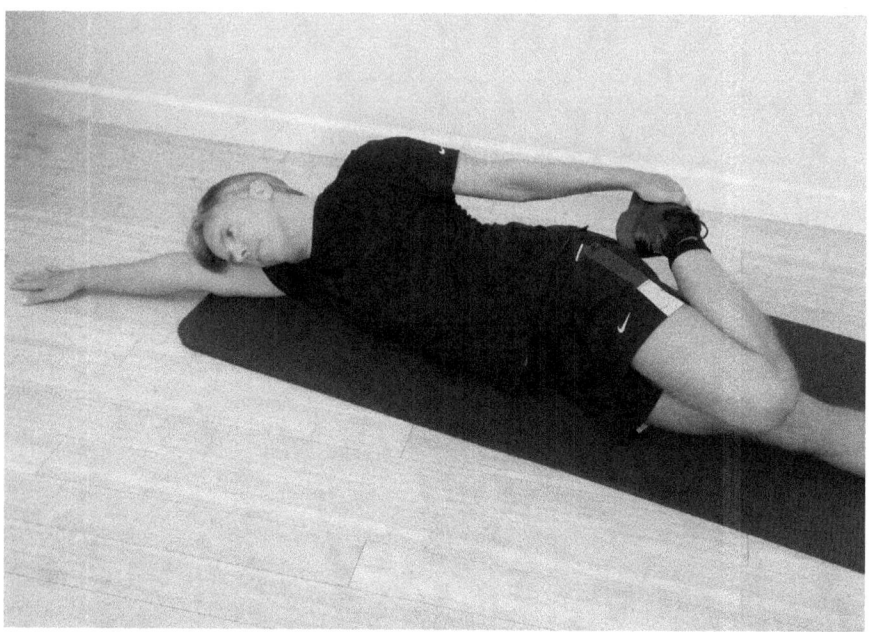

Lie on your side and rest your head on your extended arm. Bring the top foot up until you can grasp it. Hold for 15-30 seconds and repeat 3 times for each leg. You will have to roll over to stretch your other leg.

3. Standing Thigh and Back of Leg Stretch

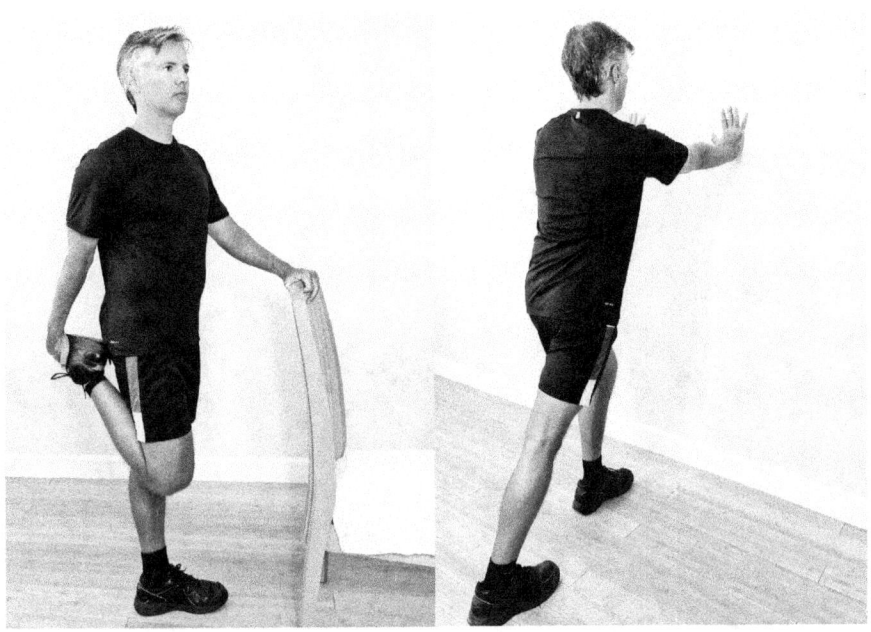

Thigh Stretch: Using a chair for balance, stand straight and bring your foot up until you can grasp it. Make sure your foot is directly behind your rear, not out to the side. Hold for 15-30 seconds and repeat 3 times for each leg.

Back of Leg Stretch: Stand straight just over arms' length away from a wall. Lean forward and place your palms flat against the wall. Bend your left leg and kick your right leg back. With both feet flat on the floor, lower your bent left leg until you feel the stretch in your right calf and thigh. Hold for 15-30 seconds and repeat 3 times for each leg. Do not force your right foot down to the floor or bounce on it. Ease up on the stretch if you feel any pain or extreme tightness.

4. Lean Forward Back Stretch

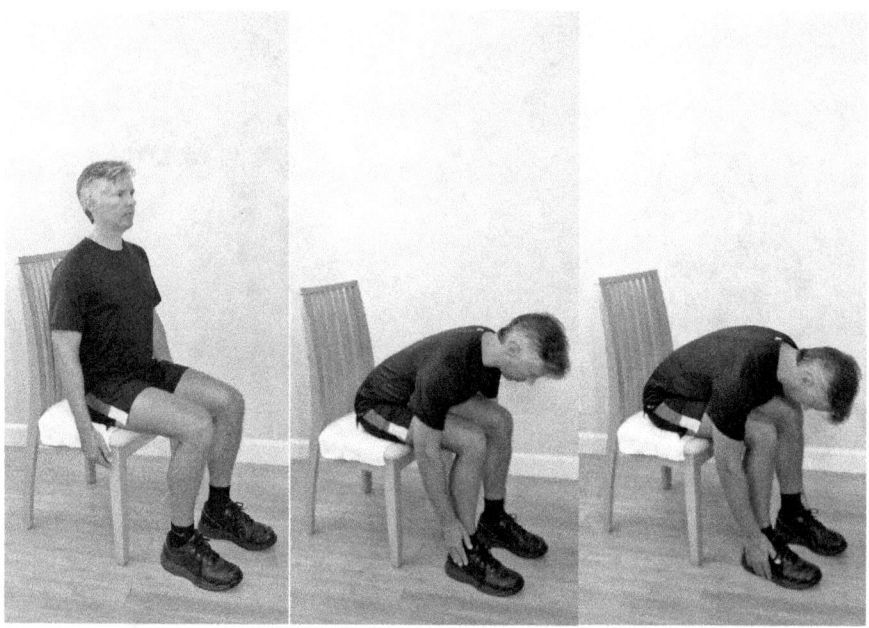

Sit straight on the front edge of a chair. Keeping your neck and back straight, slowly lean forward from your hips. Reach your calves, then relax your neck and reach your ankles. Exhale as you straighten your neck and back again and rise back up. Perform this stretch slowly 3 times.

5. Upper Back and Chest Stretch

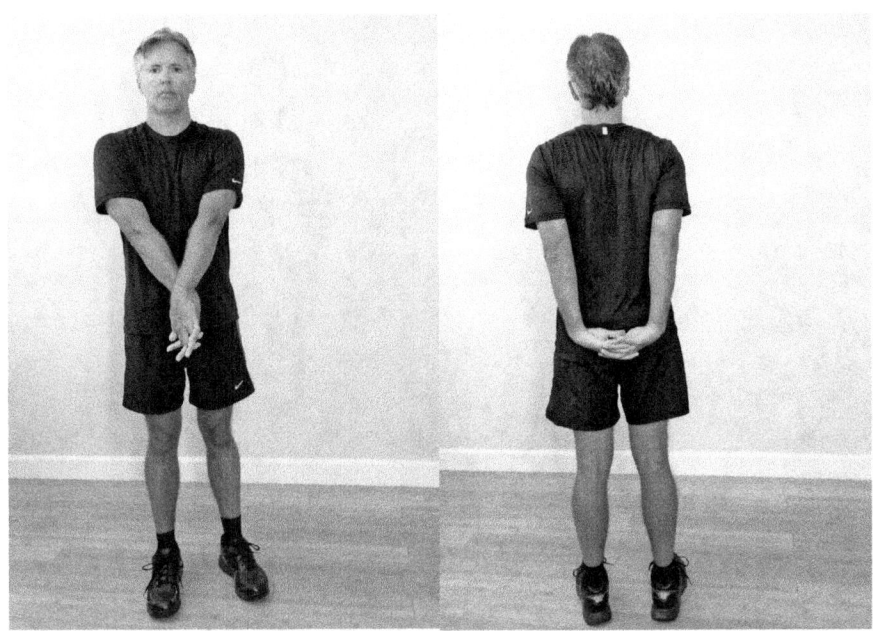

Upper Back: Standing straight, clasp your hands in a hand-over hand fashion with interlaced fingers. With straight arms, pull your shoulders forward. You will feel the stretch in your upper back. Hold for 15-30 seconds and repeat 3 times.

Chest Stretch: Standing straight, clasp your hands with interlaced fingers behind you and lower your hands as far as comfortable while expanding your chest to feel the stretch. Hold for 15-30 seconds and repeat 3 times.

6. Chest and Neck Stretch

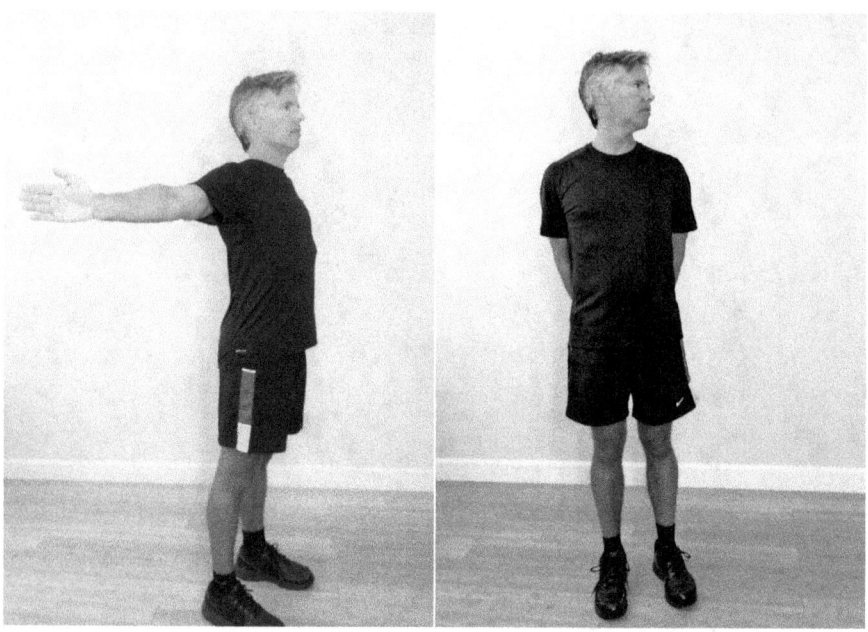

Chest Stretch: Standing or sitting straight, palms facing forward and arms at shoulder height, move your arms back as far as is comfortable. Hold for 15-30 seconds and repeat 3 times.

Neck Stretch: Sitting or standing straight, turn your head to one side until you feel a stretch. Hold for 15-30 seconds and repeat 3 times looking right and left. Be gentle and do not apply force to turn your head beyond a comfortable range.

INTERMEDIATE STRETCHES

These stretches are for people who have achieved a reasonable level of fitness and who do not have health, mobility or balancing issues.

Perform each of these stretches three times and hold them for 15-30 seconds. **If you have had neck, back, hip, or knee surgery, absolutely get your physician's permission before stretching or exercising.**

1. Whole Body Stretch

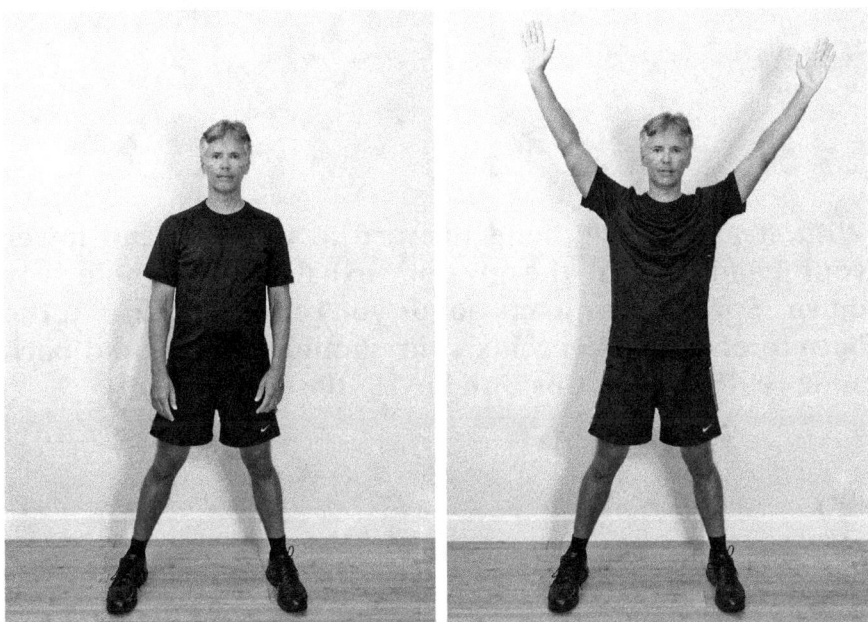

Stand straight with feet spread just beyond shoulder-width apart. Raise your hands and reach toward the sky to stretch your upper torso. Take a deep breath and...

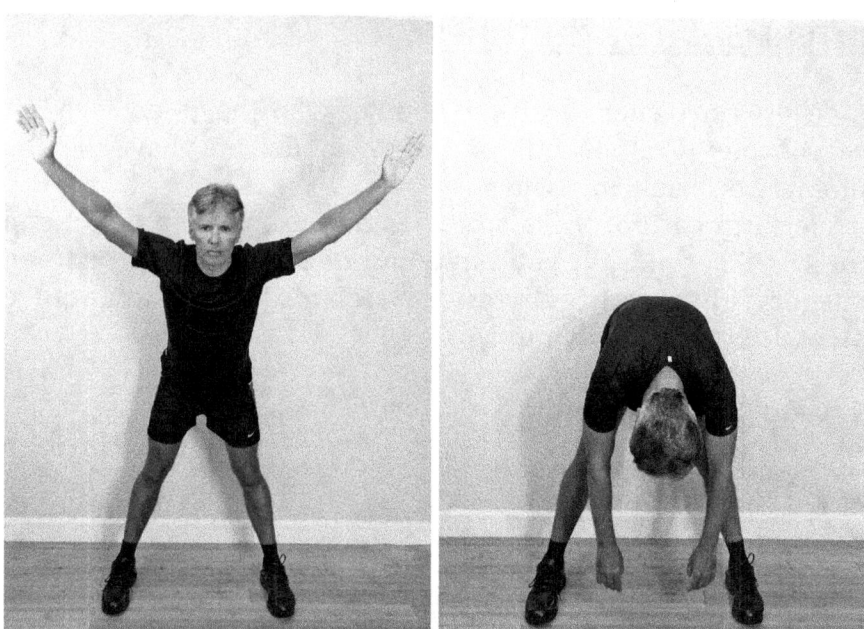

With straight back, bend forward at the hips and lower your head toward the ground, exhaling the whole way down. Spread your arms out as you're descending. At the bottom of the move, relax your shoulder, arms, and back and breathe in this position for 15-30 seconds...

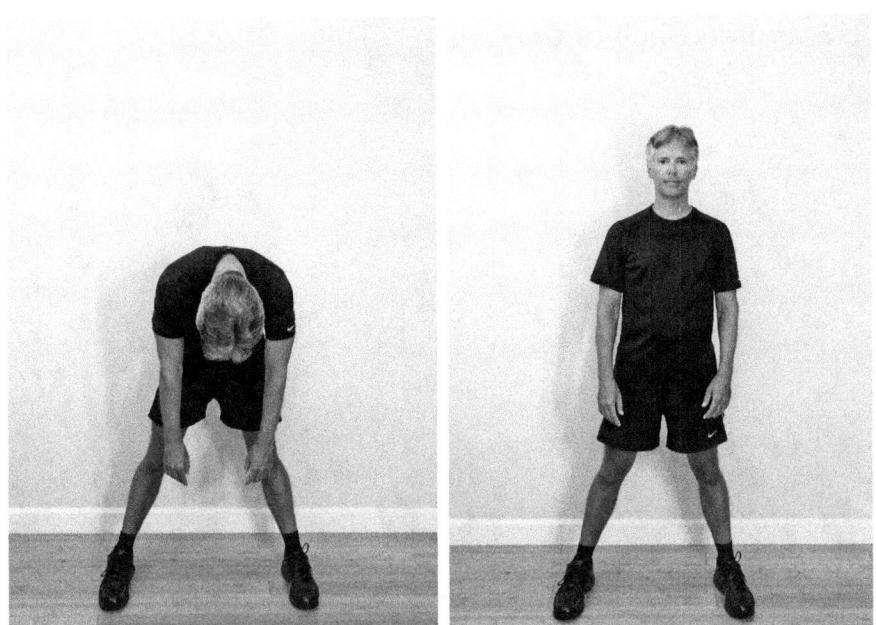

Then slowly roll your back up – instead of having a straight back -- to the starting position. Repeat 5 times.

2. Standing Back of the Leg and Thigh Stretch

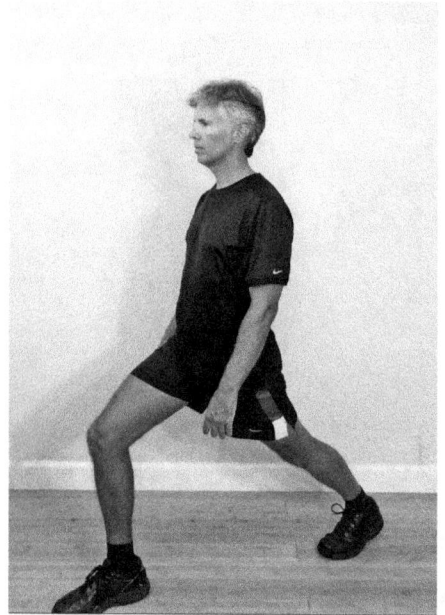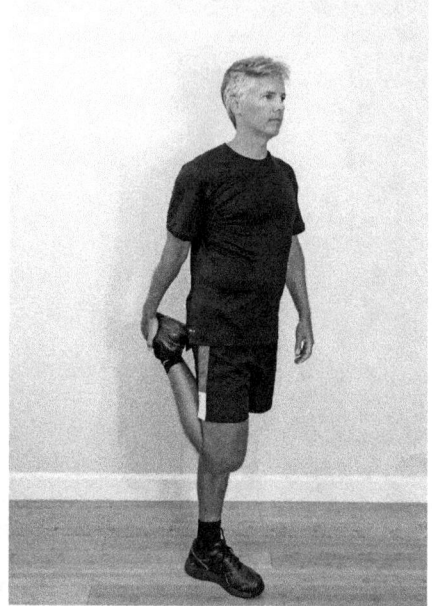

Back of the Leg: Use a chair for balance if necessary. Stand straight, step forward and bend your forward knee while keeping your back leg straight with your heel off the floor. Ease your weight onto the back leg to stretch the back of the leg. Do not force the back foot down by applying weight or bouncing. The stretch will be felt in the front of the thigh and calf. Hold for 15-30 seconds and repeat 3 times for each leg.

Thigh: Use a chair for balance if necessary. Standing straight, lift a foot directly behind you until you can grasp your shoe. Hold the stretch for 15-30 seconds and repeat 3 times for each leg. Do not flare your leg out at the hip. The foot has to be directly behind your rear for the stretch to work.

3. Knee and Hip Stretch

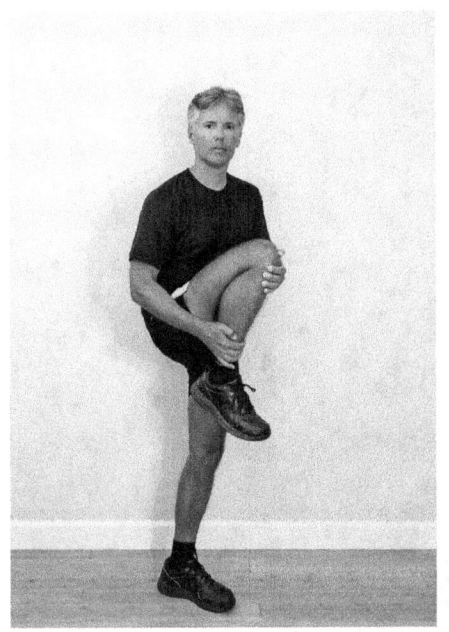 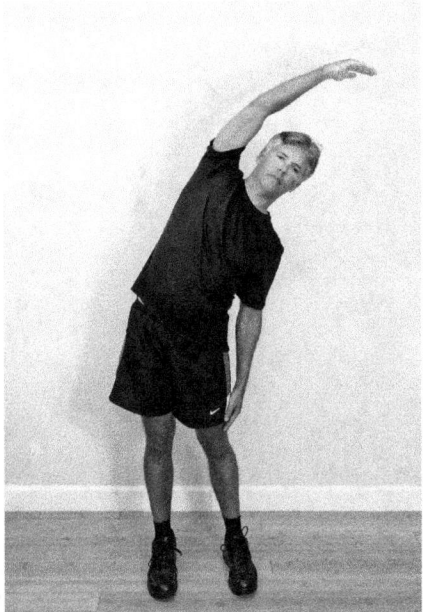

Knee: This is a difficult stretch that requires excellent balance. Skip it if you are unable to stand safely in this position. Stand straight and lift one leg slowly up straight in front of you. Stop when you are able to grasp your knee and ankle. Gently pull your leg up slightly to enhance the stretch. Hold for 15-30 seconds and repeat 3 times for each leg.

Hip: Stand straight, lift your hand over your head, and arch to the opposite side until you feel the stretch in your hip and the side of your upper torso. Hold for 15-30 seconds and repeat 3 times for each side.

4. Upper Back and Chest Stretch

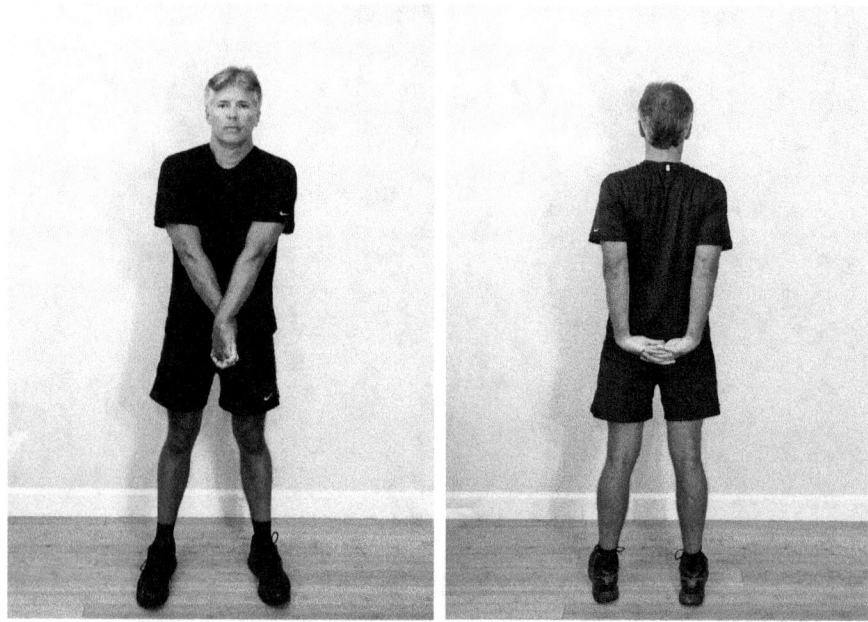

Upper Back: Standing straight, clasp your hands in a hand-over hand fashion with interlaced fingers. With straight arms, pull your shoulders forward. You will feel the stretch in your upper back. Hold for 15-30 seconds and repeat 3 times.

Chest Stretch: Standing straight, clasp your hands with interlaced fingers behind you and lower your hands as far as is comfortable while expanding your chest to feel the stretch. Hold for 15-30 seconds and repeat 3 times.

5. Shoulder Stretch

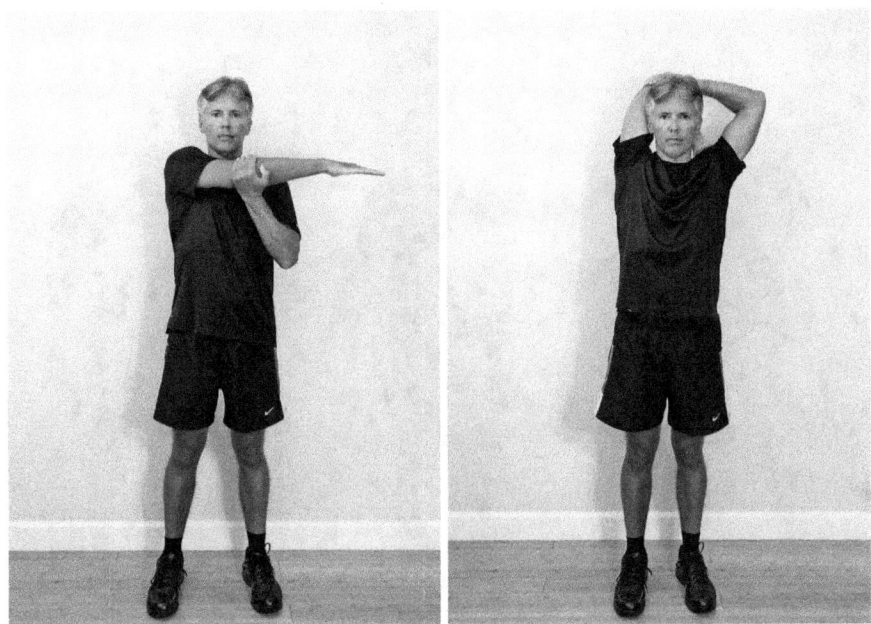

Stand straight, bring a straight arm up to shoulder length and grab your elbow. Pivot the straight arm in toward your body and feel the stretch in your shoulder. Hold for 15-30 seconds.

Reach the same arm straight up next to your head, bend at the elbow, and put your hand on the opposite shoulder. Use your other hand to gently pull the elbow in toward your head. When you just start to feel the stretch, hold it there. Do not pull harder to get a greater stretch. Hold for 15-30 seconds and repeat 3 times for each shoulder.

6. Neck Stretch

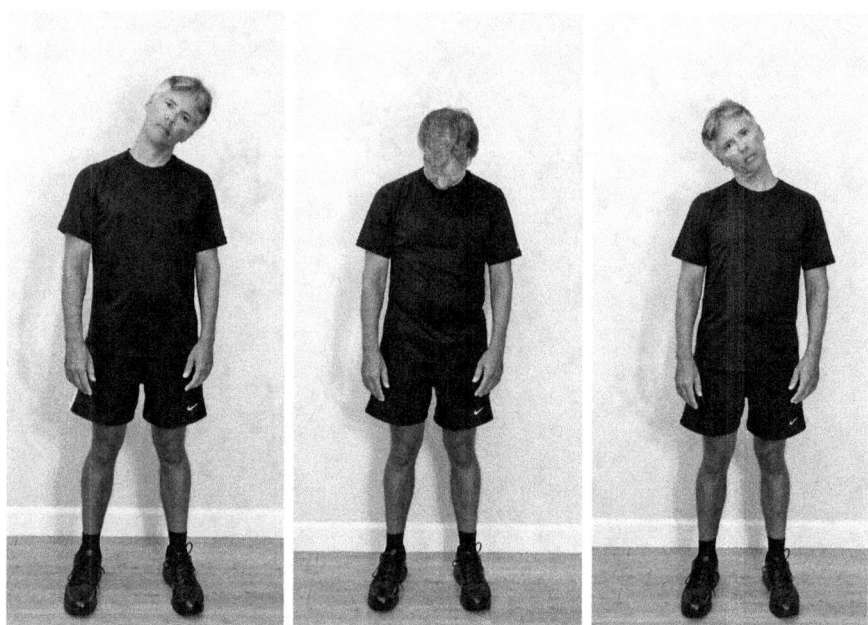

Stand straight with shoulders relaxed and arms hanging by your side. Tilt your head to the right and hold for 15-30 seconds. Do not lift your shoulders. Tilt your head forward and hold for 15-30 seconds. Then tilt your head to the left and hold for 15-30 seconds. Repeat three times in each position. Absolutely do not perform neck circles as these can damage the vertebrae in your neck.

TREATING POST-WORKOUT SORENESS

Post-workout soreness is a common problem for people just beginning a fitness program and experienced hands who increases their exercise intensity. Once your body gets used to the new physical challenges you're throwing at it, the soreness will go away.

In the meantime, making an effort to alleviate the soreness is worth it as it will keep you from giving up on your fitness program. The following steps should help:

> Gradually introduce your body to exercise or extra intensity to head off the soreness.

> Alternate aerobic exercise and strength training days to give the muscles involved in each adequate time to recover.

> For the first 48 hours, apply ice wrapped in a cloth to the affected area for up to 20 minutes at a time.

> After the icing period is over, apply heat in the form of warm to hot wet towels to restore blood flow and loosen the affected area.

> Take hot showers or baths to relax tight muscles.

> Get a massage.

> Take a doctor-approved analgesic – aspirin, ibuprofen, or naproxen – to reduce inflammation.

> Take a few days off between exercise sessions and resume working out when the soreness is gone.

If the soreness persists for more than three days or you're concerned that the problem is more serious than regular muscle soreness, do not hesitate to contact your doctor.

10 TIPS FOR OTHER AEROBIC EXERCISES

Walking and running are just two of dozens of aerobic activities that will improve your cardiovascular health. Following are helpful general tips for other popular activities people use to fulfill the aerobic exercise requirement. The trick to staying in the game is finding activities that you truly enjoy so you are inspired to continue to work out with consistency and enthusiasm.

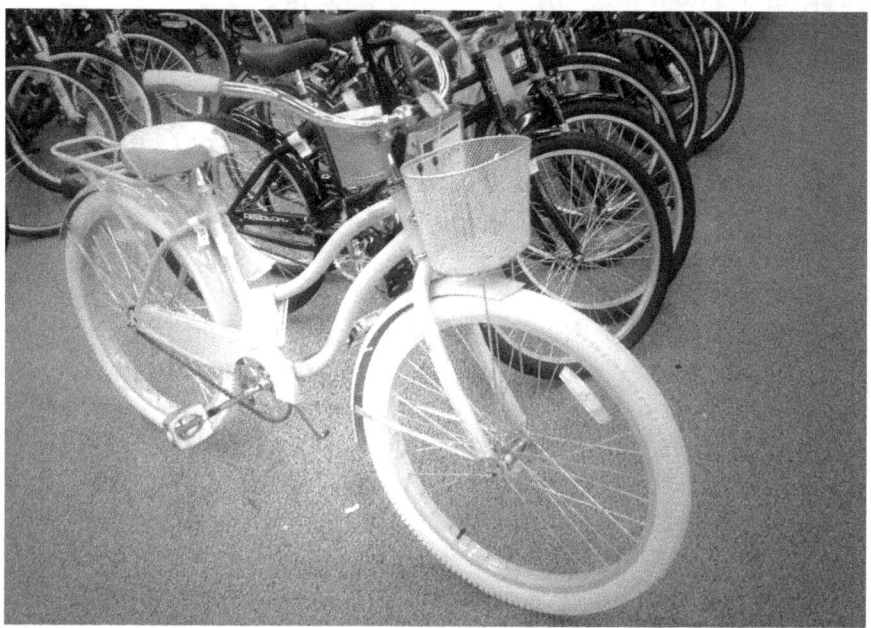

CYCLING

Riding a bike is a healthy, low-impact exercise that fills the lungs with fresh air and gets the heart pumping. Here are some tips to help you get started:

1. **Choose a bike that's appropriate for your intended course.** There are many kinds of bikes to choose from, including racing bikes for street use, mountain bikes for trails, and cruising bikes for casual touring.

2. **Purchase a bike appropriate for your size.** Bikes come in different sizes to accommodate different heights and leg lengths. Most bikes will have tags that tell you the type of body build they're intended to serve.

3. **Consider riding posture.** Racing and mountain bikes require you to lean forward, putting a great deal of weight on your shoulders, arms, elbows, and wrists. If you don't have enough strength to handle the weight or you have shoulder, arm, elbow, or wrist issues, consider purchasing a cruising bike that allows you to sit upright and lightly grip the handlebars or a recumbent bike that allows you to pedal from a reclining position.

4. **Adjust your seat.** For safety and comfort, your seat should be adjusted high enough that your leg is 80-90 percent extended on the down pedal.

5. **Purchase a gel seat or gel riding shorts.** Even cushioned bike seats can be hard on your rear end. If you experience pain, don't give up. To alleviate the pain, try a gel seat, gel seat cover, or gel riding shorts.

6. **Wear a helmet and bright clothing.** Bike accidents are among the leading cause of sports-related emergency room admissions. Reduce the risk by wearing a bike helmet at all times along with bright clothing to make you more visible to drivers.

7. **Equip your bike with reflectors and lights.** Bikes, just like cars, need reflectors and lights to be visible in low light situations or at night. A white front light and red tail light will substantially increase your visibility.

8. **Follow the rules of the road.** Flowing in the same direction as traffic, staying in bike lanes or at the side of the road, and obeying traffic signs and signals are a must.

9. **Don't assume drivers can see you.** In this dangerous day of drivers being distracted by cell phone calls and texting, it's more important than ever that you never assume motorists can see you. Always assume they can't and ride defensively. Also, beware of drivers backing out of driveways, signaling a left when they mean a right, and opening doors ahead of you. These are among the most common causes of collisions.

10. **Ride with a buddy, let people know your route, and bring a cell phone, ID, health insurance card, cash, and a tire repair kit.** Bike riders generally don't stay in their own neighborhoods, which means they have to be prepared for emergency situations and accidents. Before you go out, practice using your tire repair kit and placing the chain where it belongs so you don't have to learn how to make repairs by the side of the road.

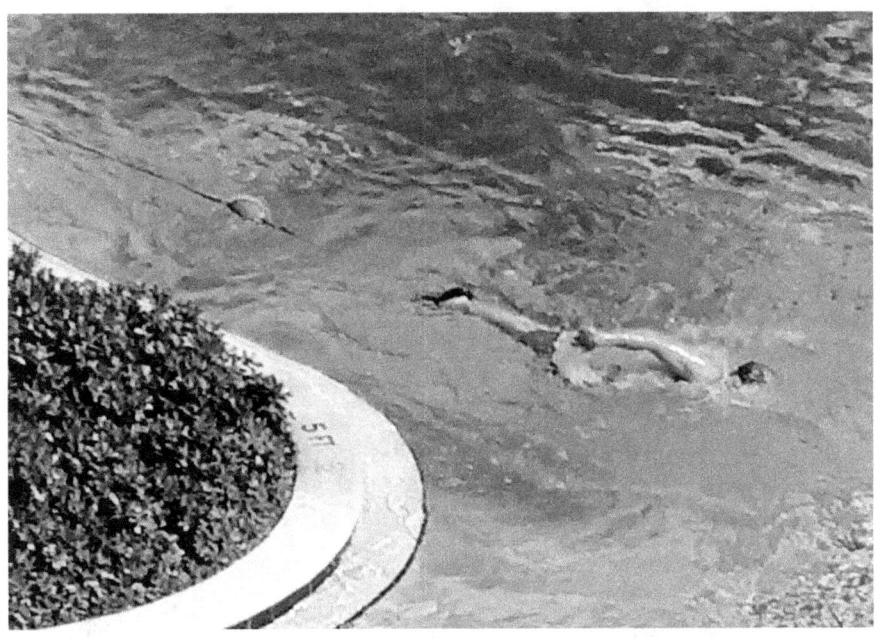

SWIMMING

Swimming is a super low impact exercise that, when performed correctly, builds cardiovascular health and upper body strength. It's excellent for people with muscle, bone, and joint problems. Here are some swimming tips to help you get started:

1. **Take lessons.** Swimming lanes is a repetitive exercise that must be performed with proper form to yield the greatest health benefits for the effort. Taking lessons is a great way to ensure you're swimming with correct form to get the most out of every session.

2. **Be patient.** Learning good technique requires controlled breathing and being aware of each movement that must be made in the right order to propel your body through the water. If you're an experienced, self-taught swimmer, you may have to break some bad habits. Be patient, put in the time to

develop correct form, and you will see marked improvement over time.

3. **Wear goggles and earplugs.** This essential equipment will protect your eyes and ears from damage and infection from prolonged exposure to water.

4. **Warm up before you get in the pool.** Make sure your muscles are warmed up by taking a five to ten minute walk before you get in the pool.

5. **Stretch after each exercise session.** Performing one of the stretching routines that appear earlier in this chapter will ensure that your muscles are limber the next time you work out.

6. **Never swim alone.** People in distress can drown in less than two minutes. If you have a muscle cramp or another medical emergency, you need someone there to help you to safety.

7. **Never swim while impaired.** Alcohol or drugs can dull your senses, which is a dangerous state of mind when you're immersed in water. When in doubt, stay out.

8. **Swim near a lifeguard.** A lifeguard is your best protection in an emergency.

9. **Watch out for rip currents.** Rip currents are powerful rivers of water that run away from the shoreline. If you feel a tug out to sea, get out of the water. If you get stuck in a rip current, don't panic. Swim parallel to shore to get out of it, then swim in to shore. If you can't swim free of the rip current, ride it out, it will eventually weaken, then swim diagonally back into shore.

10. **Take group classes.** If swimming lanes is too monotonous for you, consider taking a water aerobics

class to spice things up and increase opportunities to socialize.

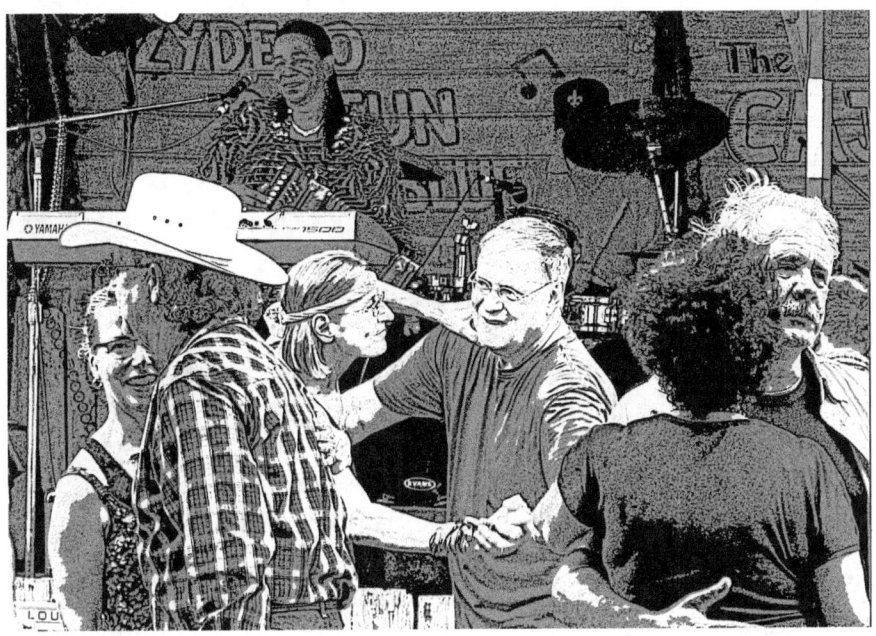

DANCING

Dancing is a terrific whole-body and mind exercise. It builds cardiovascular health, upper and lower body strength, and balance and coordination, while bolstering mental alertness as you learn to execute new moves. Social interaction during dance sessions is also good for warding off depression. These tips will help you hit the floor:

1. **Take classes.** Local high schools, community colleges, and private continuing education schools often hold affordable dance classes.

2. **Start simple.** Dancing might look natural but it doesn't come naturally to most people. The waltz is a great style to take up first. Learning to keep your feet moving to the 1-2-3 beat and then adding advanced arm moves will give you a solid basis for more advanced dance

forms, such as swing, salsa, and other ballroom styles.

3. **Be patient.** At first, learning how to dance – interpreting the beat into actual motion – is like learning how to walk all over again. Your brain has to build new links all the way down to your feet. Investing the time, effort, and patience to do it well pays off.

4. **Practice.** After every class, make sure to practice what you've learned. Practice is the best way to reinforce each lesson until you get it right.

5. **Break each move down into tiny movements.** Even the simplest dance requires people to perform many movements in the right sequence. Breaking each move down and performing it in slow motion, then gradually speeding it up, is the most productive approach.

6. **Get used to dancing in public.** Dancing is a spectator sport. Practice your moves at home, and, when you get them down, take your act on the road. Go to a festival, dance hall, or club and dance on the sidelines until you're comfortable in the spotlight.

7. **Socialize.** Knowing how to dance is a great ice-breaker. People are always looking for a competent partner. When you're ready, invite people to dance with you. Just realize few people dance with exactly the same skill and style, so be open to accommodating them.

8. **Be supportive of your partner.** Dancing comes easier to some people than others, and learning how to dance can be a very emotional experience. Being supportive of your partner is critical throughout the learning process. Non-constructive criticism, frustration, and anger is destructive to the process.

9. **Learn from others.** Every style of dance has dozens of

moves. When you go out, watch others dance and don't be afraid to ask them how to execute a move you admire during a break. Most dancers are very social, and they will gladly show you their methods.

10. **Have fun!** Dancing is one of the most enjoyable total body exercises. The really neat thing is once you get in the groove, you'll forget it's exercise and see it more as an expression of joy.

FINAL THOUGHTS

Aerobic exercise revitalizes the body, mind, and spirit. Taking up aerobic exercise and staying with it will reinvigorate your life and open more doors than it closes.

Many people who take part in aerobic exercise, especially walking and running, overlook the importance of strength training in their quest to develop whole-body fitness. Leaving out this piece of the puzzle is a serious mistake.

Walking and running do nothing to develop upper body strength. Taking the time to train with resistance, promotes muscle, bone, and joint health throughout the body, which gives people a solid foundation for aerobic activities.

We'll take a detailed look at strength training in the next chapter.

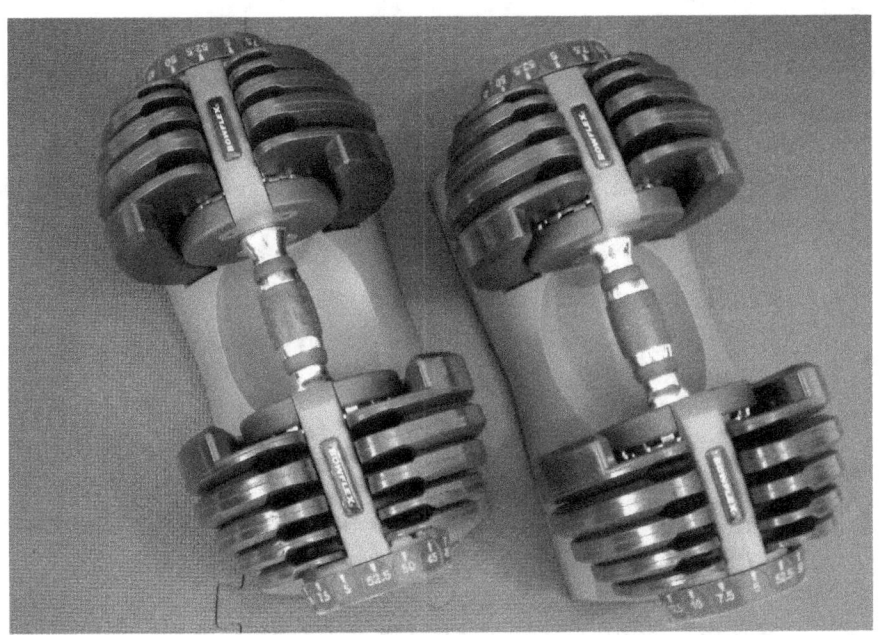

4 STRENGTH TRAINING

<u>Strength Training Requirement</u>:

> ➤ **Two or more sessions a week on non-consecutive days of muscle-strengthening activity.**

> ➤ **Selected exercises must address the major muscle groups – legs, hips, back, abdomen, chest, shoulders and arms.**

When we think of strength training, we often imagine enormous Olympic weight lifters straining under barbells loaded with hundreds of pounds of weight or ripped athletes spending hours every day at the gym sculpting their bodies to perfection. Fortunately, to benefit from strength training, we don't have to battle gargantuan amounts of weight or dedicate our entire lives to the gym.

In fact, for people seeking whole-body fitness – muscle

strength and tone – straining under weights and working out for hours a day is not only not necessary, it can actually be harmful, leading to fatigue and debilitating neck, shoulder, back, hip and knee injuries. You are much better off taking a measured and intelligent approach to strength training with the objective of becoming more fit by:

> Challenging your body to move resistance with proper form to get the maximum benefit from an exercise while minimizing the risk of injury.

> Only taking on as much weight or other form of resistance as you can safely handle while maintaining complete control throughout an entire exercise repetition and set (8-12 repetitions).

> Being careful not to strain, jerk, or contort your body to move a weight or other form of resistance, which will protect you from being injured or experiencing uneven development.

> Making sure that whenever you cannot handle a weight or other form of resistance with proper form and control, you reduce the amount of resistance.

> Being careful not to over train muscles to the point where you suffer fatigue, which will put you at risk of injury during subsequent workouts.

When you read these tips, you can see that they are common sense in theory and practice, yet they are often the first rules forgotten when people actually begin a strength training session. Too often strength training and ego become intertwined and people set themselves up for failure and injury. Don't be one of them. Challenge your body but treat it gently, and it will remain strong for years to come. *(Check out the Fitness category on Xeniors.com for the latest information regarding strength training.)*

Also, many women, especially, are concerned that strength training will cause them to build too much muscle mass. If you're one of them, relax. You would have to lift a tremendous amount of weight every day to yield that result. Follow the advice in this book and you'll get stronger and sleeker, not bulkier.

GET YOUR PHYSICIAN'S PERMISSION

The first thing you need to do BEFORE beginning a strength training program is **GET YOUR PHYSICIAN'S PERMISSION!**

While extremely healthy, strength training exercise increases the stress load on your body, including your blood vessels, muscles, joints, tendons, and bones. You need to make sure that you can work out without causing harm.

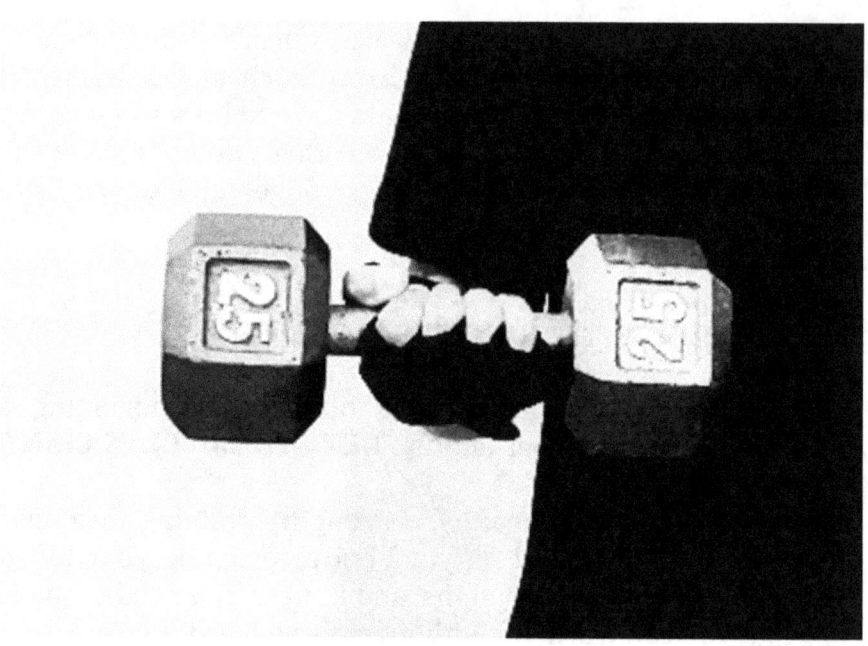

CHOOSE YOUR STRENGTH TRAINING LOCATION

Once you get your physician's permission to exercise, you need to decide where you are going to work out. The two main choices are at a gym or at home. Both can be equally productive but there are differences.

Gym

Exercising at a gym is beneficial for people who:

➢ Don't have room for a home gym.

➢ Like to have access to a wide variety of aerobic and strength training equipment and specialized facilities, like indoor swimming pools, tracks, and basketball courts.

➢ Enjoy working out with others.

➢ Want to take group classes, such as yoga, step aerobics, and spinning.

➢ Decide to hire a personal trainer.

➢ Are more motivated to exercise in an active work out setting.

The potential downsides of joining a gym are:

➢ Preparing to go to the gym and then actually traveling there is too great an investment of time and effort for some, which leads to failure.

➢ Gyms can be expensive, especially if you don't know how to negotiate the best deal with the manager.

➢ Gyms can be intimidating to people who are out of shape, so they never actually go or quit after a few visits.

➢ The temptation to spend more time socializing instead of working out causes bodies to cool down, increasing a the risk of injury.

With a little effort, each of these challenges can be overcome. First, before you join a gym, make sure you're truly committed to working out. The investment of time and effort to get to the gym is actually quite minimal if you are enthusiastic about exercise.

Second, before you choose a gym to join, tour a few and take advantage of the free week-long memberships most gyms offer. Also, make sure to get accurate cost estimates in writing that reflect initiation dues, membership dues, monthly fees and any other additional costs. Once you have the numbers, you'll be in a stronger position to negotiate with the manager. In many cases, they will give you a better deal than their published rates.

Third, if "gym-phobia" is a problem, identify why you find gyms intimidating and deal with the issue head on. Often newcomers have an over-inflated impression that everyone is watching and judging them when they first attend a gym. Certainly people take notice when someone new walks through the door, but, in most cases, they get back to their workout. After the first couple of weeks of regular attendance, they'll see you as a regular and familiarity will soon lead to friendships.

That said, experienced gym-goers know every gym has a few arrogant gym rats who, like elementary school bullies, look down their noses at people who aren't as fit as they are. Fortunately, they are never the majority, and you shouldn't allow them to control your health and fitness destiny.

There are several ways to overcome gym-phobia, including: be brave and go it alone, bring a buddy, take a class to get to know others immediately, or hire a personal fitness trainer to forge friendships with people of similar ability. Soon you'll find yourself surrounded by so much positive energy the few downers will vanish into the weight pile.

Finally, always remember why you joined the gym: to improve your whole-body fitness. Commit to focusing more time on exercising and less time on socializing, at least during your core 45-minute workout. When you're through exercising, talk to your heart's content – just make sure you're not interrupting someone else's exercise session.

Home Gym

Exercising at home is beneficial for people who:

➢ Don't want to invest the time or effort to get ready and commute to a gym.

➢ Don't want to pay initiation fees, membership fees, and monthly dues.

➢ Can't get over their gym-phobia because they believe they're too out of shape to work out in a gym.

➤ Are confident they can design an effective strength training routine without the assistance of a personal trainer.

➤ Are more comfortable exercising alone or with a buddy in the comfort of their own home.

Equipping Your Home Gym

Fortunately, for those of us who prefer the convenience and affordability of working out at home, there are many affordable equipment options. *(Please visit Xeniors.com and enter the search term "home gym" to view our article on assembling a home gym, which provides specific product recommendations..)*

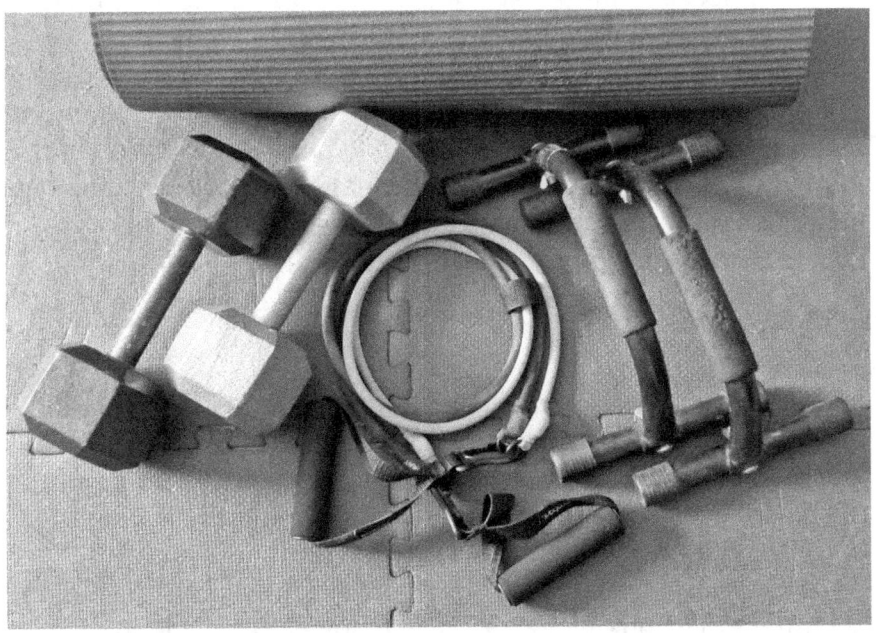

6 Home Gym Essentials

Following is a list of essential home gym equipment you'll need to exercise your major muscle groups:

1. **Rubberized floor mat** – protects your flooring from barbells and sports shoes.

2. **Yoga mat** – a cushy yoga mat will provide more comfort for exercises performed on the floor.

3. **Push-up handles** – reduce the stress on hands and wrists.

4. **Resistance bands** – a safe, portable, and light weight form of resistance that nearly everyone can use.

5. **Dumbbells** – provide the maximum range of motion with a small space requirement.

6. **A door frame mounted pull-up bar** – this is extra for experts. Pull-ups are one of the most difficult exercises, but they're extremely good for your body.

If you go the home gym route, you have to manage your gym to avoid injuring yourself and damaging your home. Remember to use the equipment according to the manufacturer's recommendations and monitor the equipment for wear and tear and replace it as needed.

Clothing

Strength training clothing should be comfortable and allow an unimpeded range of motion while you're exercising. This means it should fit well but not too tightly. At the other end of the scale, beware of clothes that hang too loosely – they could become tangled in your workout equipment.

The most important piece of clothing that too many beginners overlook is weight lifting gloves. That's too bad, too. Gloves with padded fingers and palms can prevent painful chafing, blistering, and bruising, making strength training much more enjoyable and allowing you to heft more weight. Strength training is not about suffering. Buy a pair of gloves before you start.

12 FREQUENTLY ASKED QUESTIONS

1. **Should I strength train every day?** The requirement is two or more sessions a week. Strength training every day will put you at greater risk of dropping out due to fatigue or boredom. You should only strength train every day if you are working different major muscle groups on alternating days. This will give your muscles time to recover from the last training sessions. Most people will become fit, which is the ultimate goal of exercising, if they strength train three days a week, participate in aerobic exercise three days a week, and take an entire day off once a week to allow their entire body to recover.

2. **What time of day should I strength train?** There's no set time of day all people should strength train. You should do it when you are at your strongest. Some people bound out of bed early in the morning ready to exercise, others are at their most vital at lunchtime, the afternoon, or evening.

3. **How long should I strength train?** As long as it takes to complete exercises that address every major muscle group. If you're going over 45 minutes each session, however, you're likely over training for general fitness.

4. **Should I eat before I strength train?** Strength training is more productive and enjoyable if you're not hungry. Eat a healthy meal or a snack a half hour to hour before you exercise. Just don't eat too much. Being too full while exercising is as uncomfortable as being hungry.

5. **How many exercises should I do?** That depends on how fit you are. In the beginning you might want to perform eight repetitions (complete exercise motions)

of each exercise for each major muscle group. Once your body gets stronger and you can perform 12-15 repetition of each exercise – otherwise known as a set -- you can increase the number of sets to two or three per exercise per workout session. (We'll explore this further when we discuss actual beginner and intermediate strength training routines.)

6. **How much weight or resistance should I use?** As much as you can handle with total control and proper form through an entire repetition, set, and workout session. The best way to determine how much weight or other resistance you can handle is through experimentation. For example, in the gym or at a sporting goods store, find the lightest weight you think you can handle and see if you can take it through the range of motion of an exercise with total control. If you can, and it seems too easy, go to the next higher weight. Do this until you reach the point where you feel like you have to work to complete eight repetitions with proper form and total control without contorting, jerking, or straining your body. If you can, you found your weight. It's also a good idea to purchase a weight just above and just below your target weight so you have something to use when you're feeling great or a little slow.

7. **How do I know when it's time to increase the amount of weight or resistance?** When you can complete 12-15 repetition with proper form, it's time to increase the weight. Use the same process as discussed above, but don't get too ambitious and take on more weight than you can safely handle.

8. **How should I strength train if I want to tone my muscles not build bulk?** All strength training tones muscles. To build bulk, you would have to lift an enormous amount of weight many times a week. So it's not a problem for most people exercising for general

fitness.

9. **Should I work out alone?** Ideally, no. Working with weights and other forms of resistance can lead to accidents or injury that may require the assistance of another person. The other value in working out with a buddy is they can help make sure that you're performing an exercise correctly. If you must work out alone, have a phone nearby and never, ever lift more weight than you can safely handle – especially during exercises like bench presses where you could potentially get pinned under the bar. (Using dumbbells is one way to eliminate this problem.)

10. **Is "no pain, no gain" true?** Absolutely not! The exertion of exercise – working muscles – shouldn't be described as painful. If you are experiencing pain, it could be due to performing exercises with improper form, you're injured, or your equipment is malfunctioning. When you feel pain, stop, locate the source, and change how you are performing an exercise, substitute it with another pain-free exercise that works the same muscle group, or replace the faulty equipment.

11. **Should I work out if I'm injured or ill?** Quite frankly, no. Injury and/or illness are signs that your body is in distress and needs to heal. Trying to power your way through it will only delay your recovery or lead to more injury and a lengthier recovery period. The only exception is that if one part of your body is injured but you can still work another area. For example, if you sprained your ankle, that might not preclude you from performing upper body exercises in a seated position.

12. **What should I do if I'm injured?** Stop what you're doing. Evaluate the severity of the injury. If it's serious – for example a broken bone or torn hamstring or

Achilles' tendon – seek immediate medical attention. If it's minor – an ankle sprain or muscle pull – try treating it by applying ice wrapped in a face cloth to the affected area for no more than twenty minutes at a time for up to 48 hours after the initial injury. After that, you may need to apply warm to hot wet towels to the injured area to promote blood flow and loosen and relax the muscle or tendon. Do not resume your regular exercise activities until the injured area has fully recovered. Exercising before then puts you at risk of re-injury or causing you to exercise with improper form, which can have a negative impact on the rest of your body.

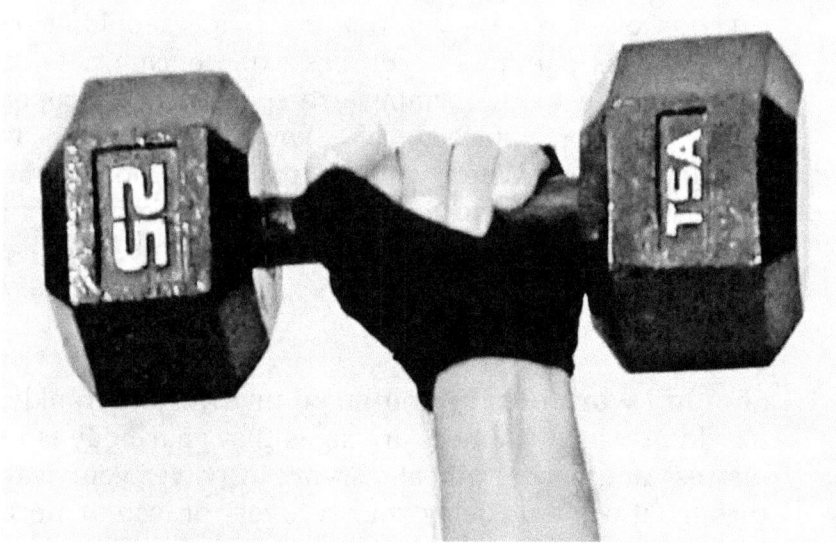

LET'S EXERCISE!

Now that you have the basics down and your physician's permission – you may want to show him or her this book for approval of specific exercises – it's time to work out. NOTE: The following warm-up, beginner strength training routine, intermediate strength training routine, and cool down and stretching sessions are featured in videos available for free on

Xeniors.com. Just visit the site and click on the Free Exercise Videos box in the right hand column.

If you don't like traditional strength training, yoga is a great alternative. Just make sure the class you take includes poses that strengthen both the upper and lower body.

WARM UP

Before you strength train, you need to spend five to ten minutes warming up your body. Starting cold is never a good idea. Your muscles need to be warmed up to extend and contract without pulling or tearing.

To prepare your body to exercise, you can either take a five to ten minute walk at your regular pace or perform the following warm-up routine.

Stretching, much to most people's surprise, is not recommended. Recent research indicates that too much stretching before exercise actually puts your body at greater risk of injury by loosening muscles and tendons to the point where they can't keep your musculoskeletal system in proper alignment during your actual workout. You'll get plenty of stretching in after your strength training session.

That said, if you have a specific problem area, such as tight Achilles' tendons, calves, or hamstrings, a little gentle stretching is a good idea. Just don't overdo it

BASIC WARM-UP ROUTINE

Perform each of the following warm-up exercises for one minute to reach a total of five minutes. Start off at a slow pace and gradually pick it up until you reach the point where you're slightly out of breath.

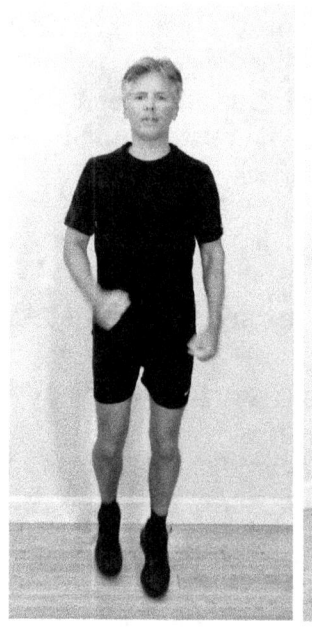 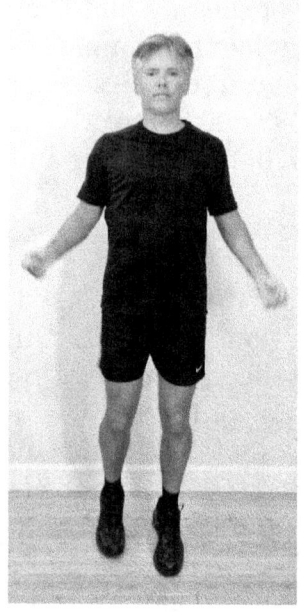 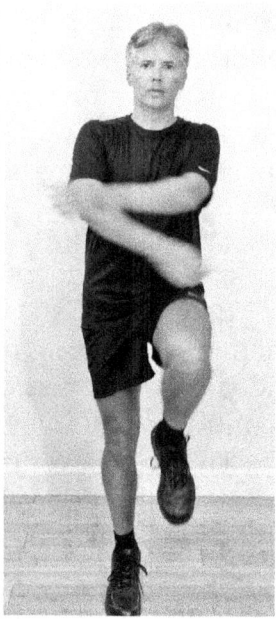

1. **Jog in place.** Go nice and easy at first and keep your arms moving. Make sure your back is straight and you relax your neck and shoulders. Also, land your feet as lightly as possible.
2. **Jump rope.** Jump an imaginary rope at an easy pace.
3. **March while hugging.** March while extending your arms out horizontally and then bring them back in and hugging your body. This warms up your neck, shoulders, and upper back.

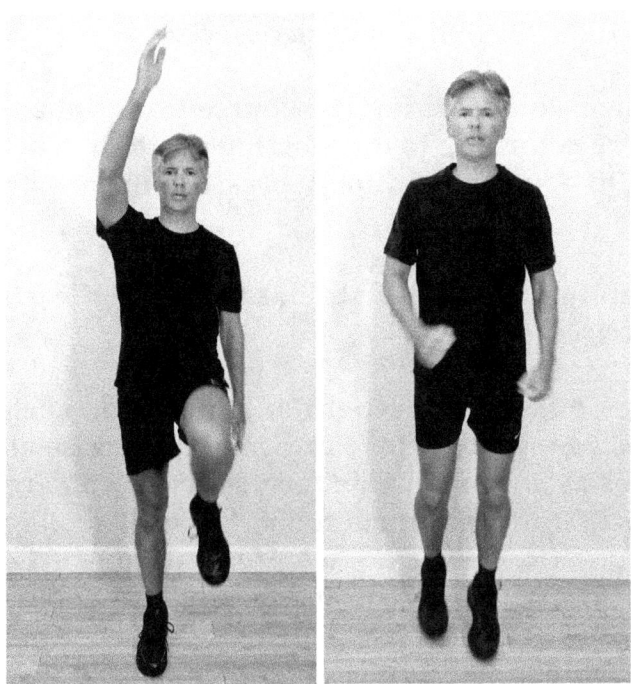

4. **March in place.** Bring your left leg and right arm up high then repeat for your right leg and left arm.
5. **Finish up jogging in place again.**

By the end of this routine, your body should be warm enough to break out in a light sweat.

CHOOSE YOUR STRENGTH TRAINING EXERCISES

At its most elemental, a strength training session is made up of specific exercises that involve lifting, lowering, pushing, and pulling some form of resistance to work each of the major muscle groups. Following are suggested exercise routines for beginners and then intermediate-level athletes. Each exercise is explained in detail. You can also visit Xeniors.com and click on our exercise video link to see how they are performed.

IMPORTANT REMINDERS! For each exercise:

➤ Exhale when you are exerting yourself and inhale when you're returning to the starting position. This will help to keep your blood pressure in a safe range.

➤ Take a minimum one minute break between each set of exercises.

➤ Realize the number or repetitions given for each exercise is a general guide. Perform the exercise as many times as is comfortable for you when you are building up strength and stamina. If you're feeling extra energetic, add a set (group of 8-12 repetitions) or two of each exercise.

➤ Stop performing any exercise that causes pain and either adjust how you are performing it or substitute another exercise that works the same major muscle group.

➤ When you are performing exercises in a standing position, do not lock your knees.

➤ Do not hesitate to contact medical professionals if you experience pain, an injury, or discomfort that causes you concern.

BEGINNER STRENGTH TRAINING ROUTINE

This beginner exercise routine is excellent for people who have never worked out before or for those with physical limitations or poor balance. Only perform the exercises your physician has approved or those that feel right to you. We'll start from the floor and work our way up.

1. Calf Raises – strengthens calves and ankles.

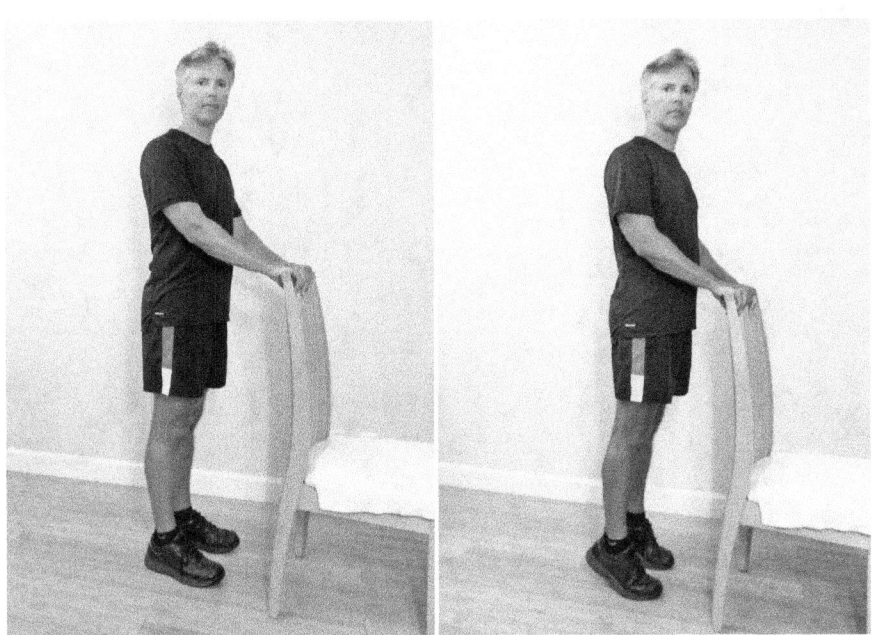

Stand straight with your hands on the back of a chair and slowly lift your heels and stand on your toes. Exhale on the way up, hold for a second or two, then inhale as you lower your heels. Repeat 8-12 times.

2. Back Leg Raise – strengthens buttocks and lower back.

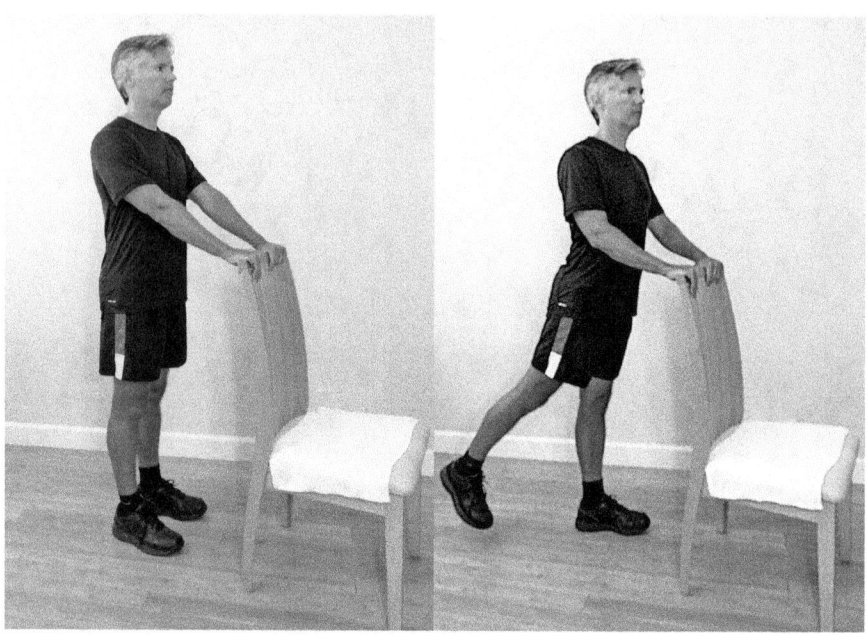

Stand straight holding onto the back of a chair. Without locking the knee you're standing on, exhale as you slowly lift a leg back without bending at the knee. Hold for a second or two, then inhale as you lower the leg to the floor. Repeat this exercise 8-12 times for each leg.

3. Leg Lift/Knee Curl – strengthens buttocks, lower leg and knee.

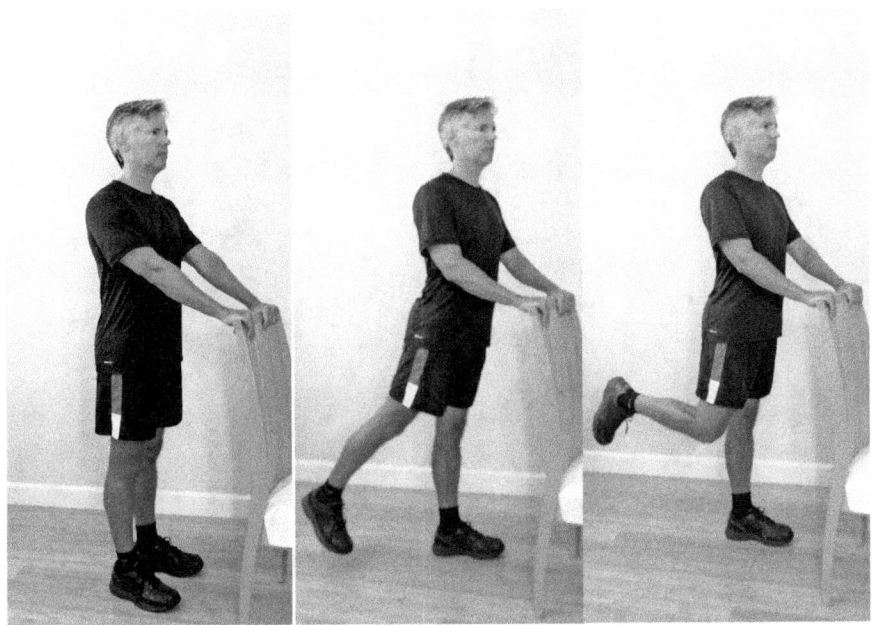

Standing straight, hold onto the back of a chair, and exhale slowly as you lift your leg behind you without bending your knee. Do not lock the knee on the leg you're standing on. Inhale, then slowly exhale and bring your heel up toward your rear end as far as you comfortably can. Hold the position for a second or two, then inhale as you lower your foot back to the floor. Repeat 8-12 times for each leg.

4. Chair stand – develops core muscles in your abdomen, and your hips and thighs.

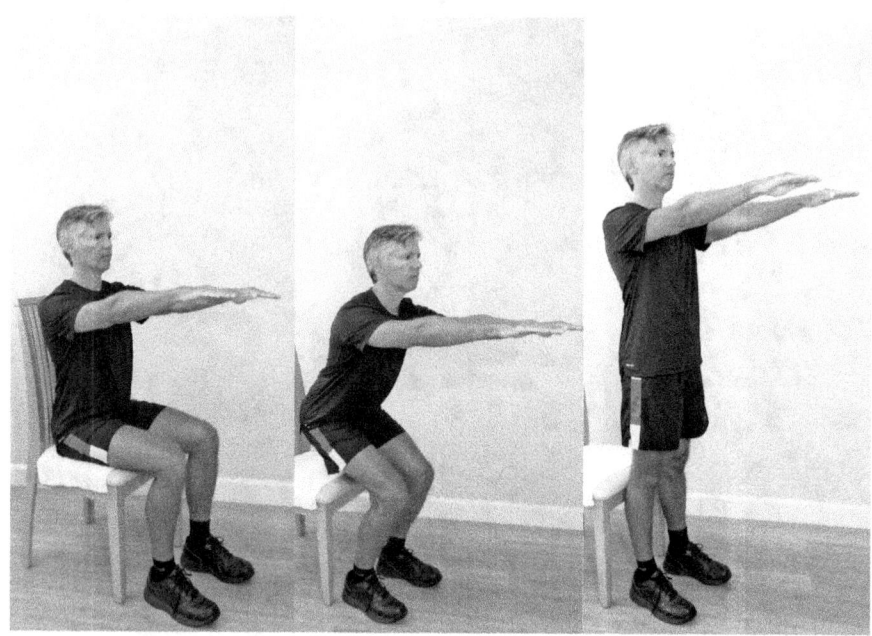

Sit straight in a chair. Extend your arms out in front of you and slowly exhale as you use your knees, thighs, hips, and abdomen muscles to rise up out of the chair. Do not lean too far forward while rising out of the chair. Inhale as you sit back down. Repeat 8-12 times.

5. Leg Extensions – strengthens thigh muscles.

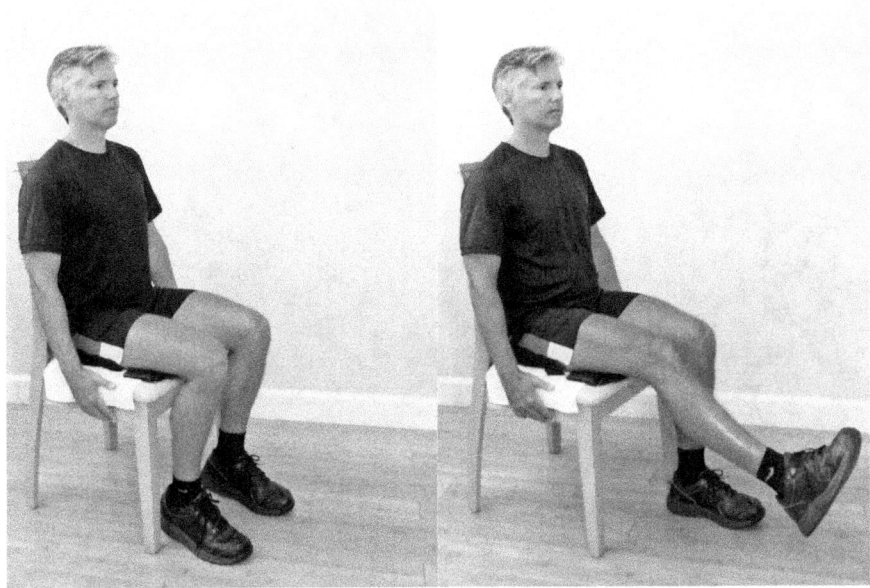

Place a towel lengthwise on the front of a chair. Sit straight in the chair with your back supported by the chair back. Exhale as you slowly lift one leg just short of locking the knee. Hold the position for a second or two then inhale as you lower the leg to the floor. Repeat 8-12 times for each leg.

6. Back Extensions – strengthens back muscles.

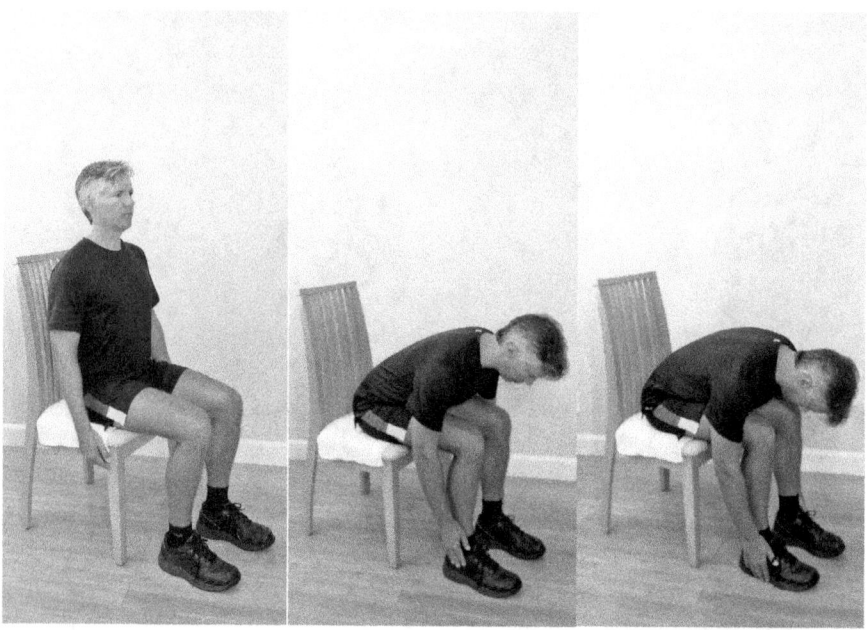

Sit straight on the front edge of a chair. Keeping your neck and back straight, exhale as you slowly lean forward at your hips. Reach your calves, then relax your neck and reach your ankles. Exhale as straighten your neck and back again and rise back up to the straight-back position. Perform this exercise slowly 3-5 times.

7. Bent Forward Row – strengthens back and shoulders.

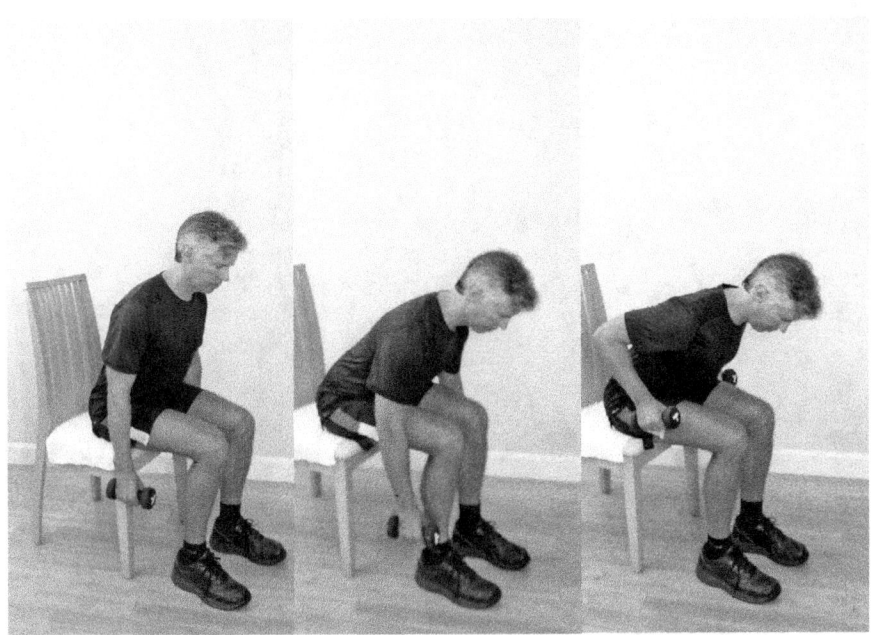

Sit straight at the forward edge of a chair holding light hand weights. With straight back and neck, slowly lean forward 45 degrees. With elbows held close to your body, exhale and slowly row the weights back using your shoulder and upper back muscles. Inhale as you lower the weights, then exhale and row them back again. Row the weights 8-12 times. Slowly return to the upright position.

8. Dumbbell Side Tilts – strengthens side abdominal muscles.

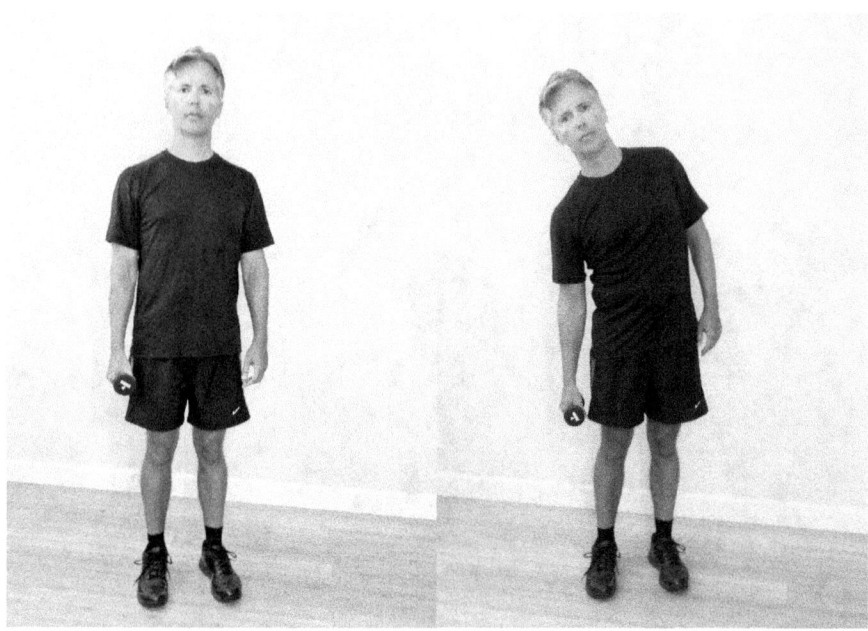

Stand straight holding a dumbbell in one hand with feet shoulder-width apart. Inhale as you tilt slowly to the side at the waist on the side holding the dumbbell. Exhale as you slowly return to the starting position. Repeat 8-12 times for each side.

9 . Wall Pushups -- strengthens chest and arms.

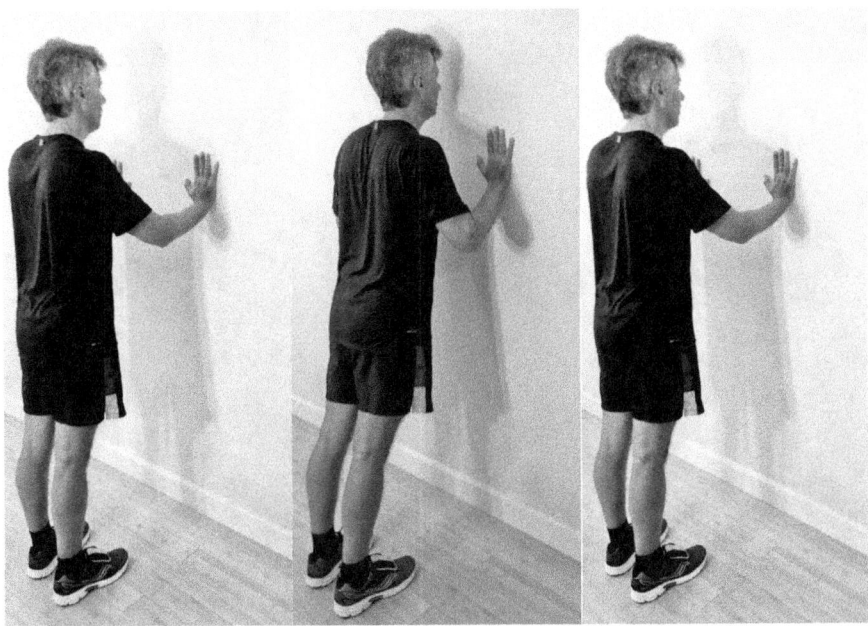

Stand arms-length (or less) away from a sturdy wall. Place your palms on the wall just below shoulder height. Inhale as you lean forward bending at the elbows. Exhale as you push slowly away from the wall. Keep your feet firmly planted and your back straight throughout the exercise. Repeat 8-12 times. Note: The further you place your feet away from the wall, the greater the resistance. Just don't go too far, or you may slip or not be able to return to an upright position.

10. Shrugs -- strengthens shoulders.

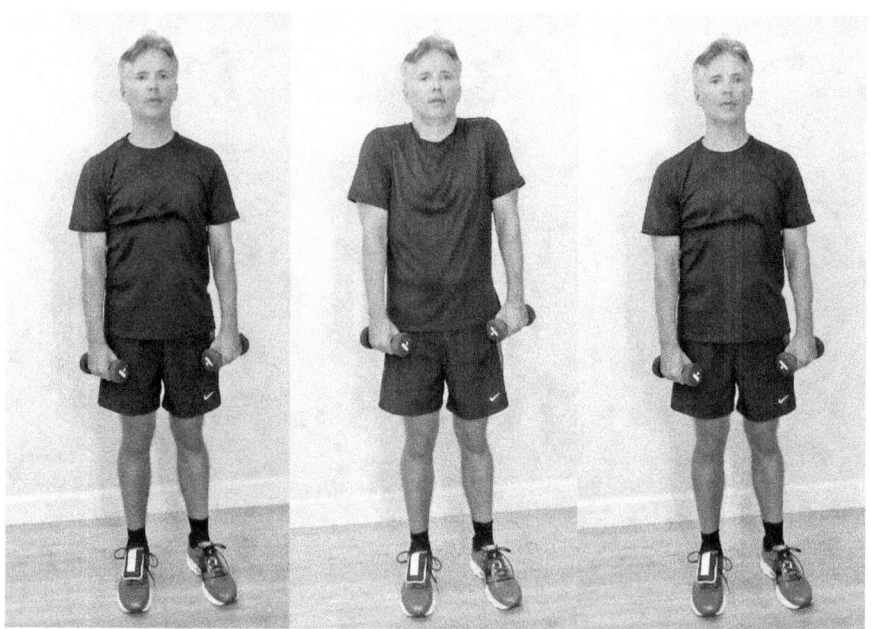

Hold weights with palms facing in toward your body. Relax your shoulders. Exhale as you raise your shoulders as far as you comfortably can. Inhale as you lower them to the starting position. Repeat 8-12 times.

Note: This exercise is excellent for people who have physical challenges that prevent them from doing the following three shoulder exercises that are more demanding.

11. Front Arm Lifts – works the shoulders.

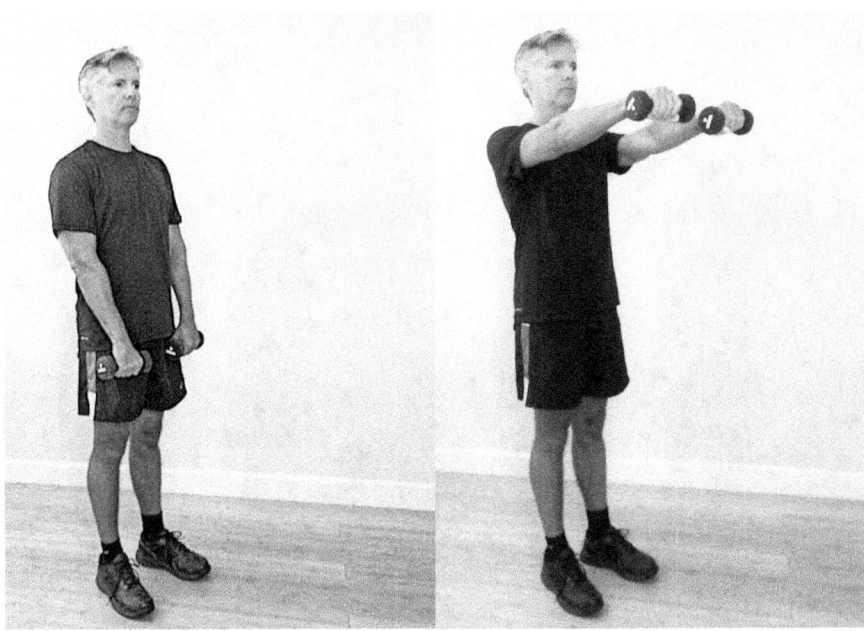

Stand straight with feet shoulder-width apart and hold two dumbbells with palms toward your body. Exhale as you slowly lift the dumbbells before you with straight arms. Inhale as you slowly lower your arms to the starting position. Repeat 8-12 times. This exercise can also be performed in a seated position.

12. Overhead Press – strengthens shoulders and arms.

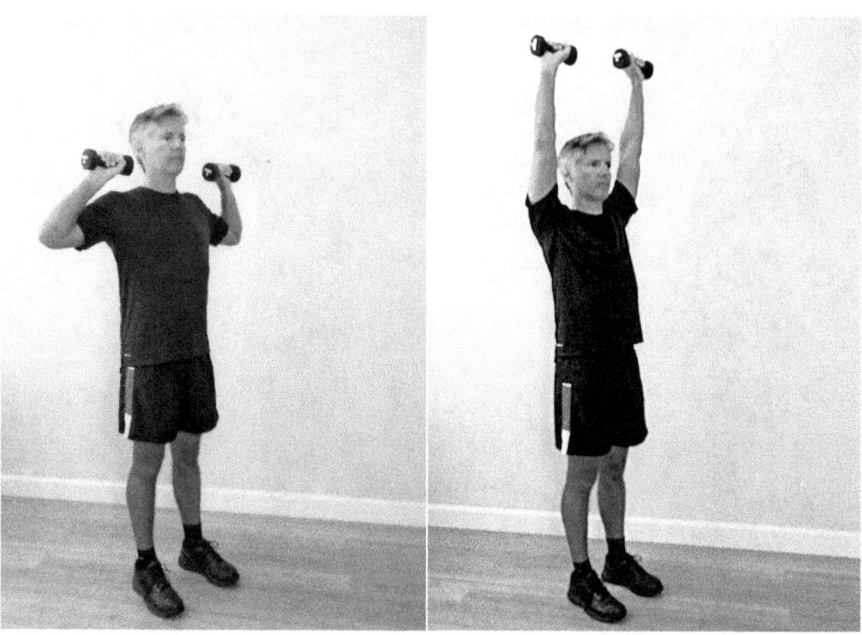

Standing with feet shoulder-width apart and holding the weights with palms forward, exhale slowly and lift the weights over your head. Inhale and lower the weights to the starting position. Repeat 8-12 times. This exercise can also be performed in a seated position.

13. Side Arm Lifts – strengthens shoulders.

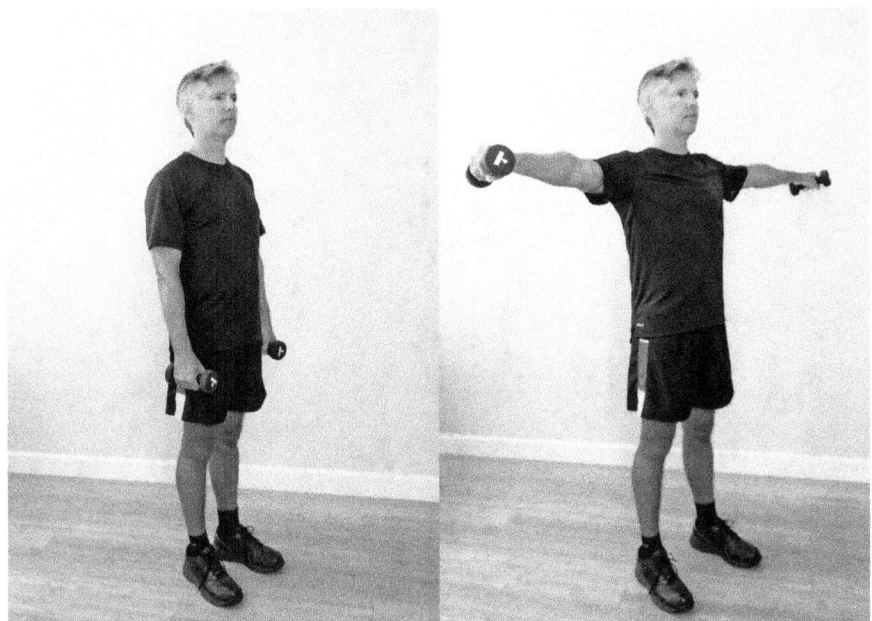

Stand straight with feet shoulder-width apart and weights held with palms in toward your body. Slowly exhale as you raise the weights with straight arms to shoulder height. Inhale as you slowly lower your arms. Repeat 8-12 times. This exercise can also be performed in a seated position.

14. Biceps Curls – strengthens the front of upper arms.

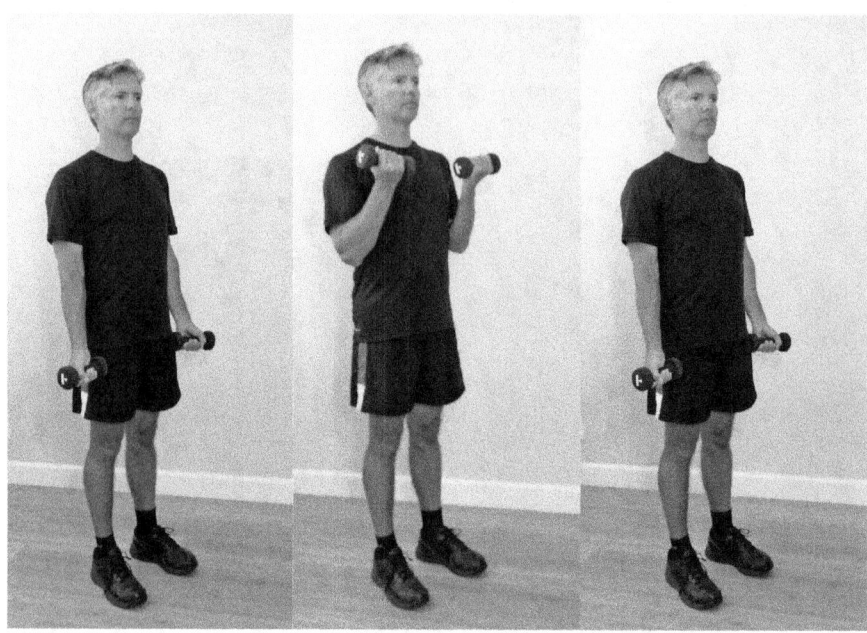

Stand straight with feet shoulder-width apart and hold your weights with palms forward. Exhale as you slowly bend your arms at the elbow and lift the weights up to your upper chest. Inhale as you slowly lower the weights to the starting position. Repeat 8-12 times.

15. Triceps Extension – works the back of upper arms.

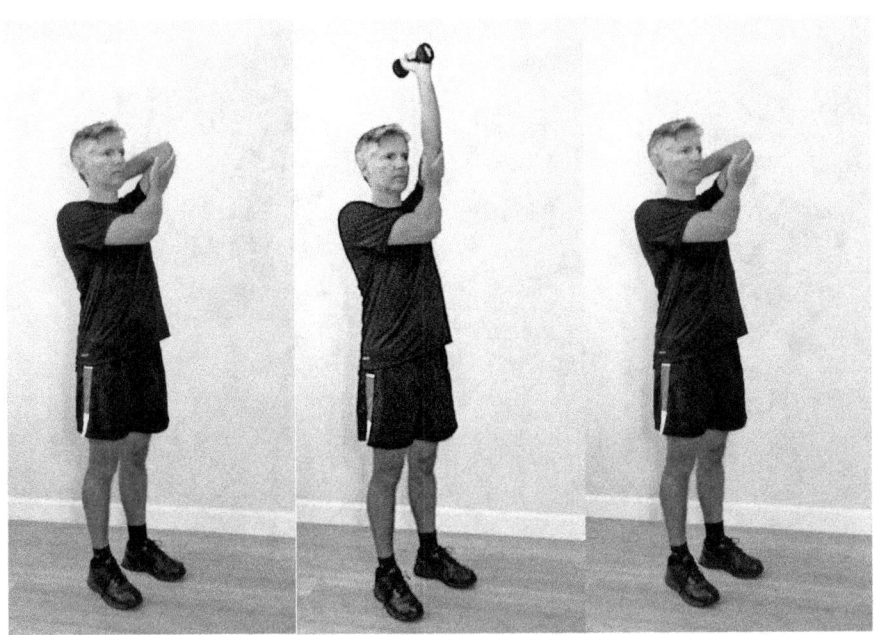

Stand straight with feet shoulder-width apart. With or without a dumbbell, raise an arm straight up, with your palm in toward your body, and brace your elbow with your other hand. Inhale as you slowly bend at the elbow and lower the weight behind you to ear level. Exhale as you raise the weight slowly back up to the starting position. Repeat 8-12 times for each arm. This exercise can also be performed in a seated position.

16. Seated Triceps Extension – works the backs of arms.

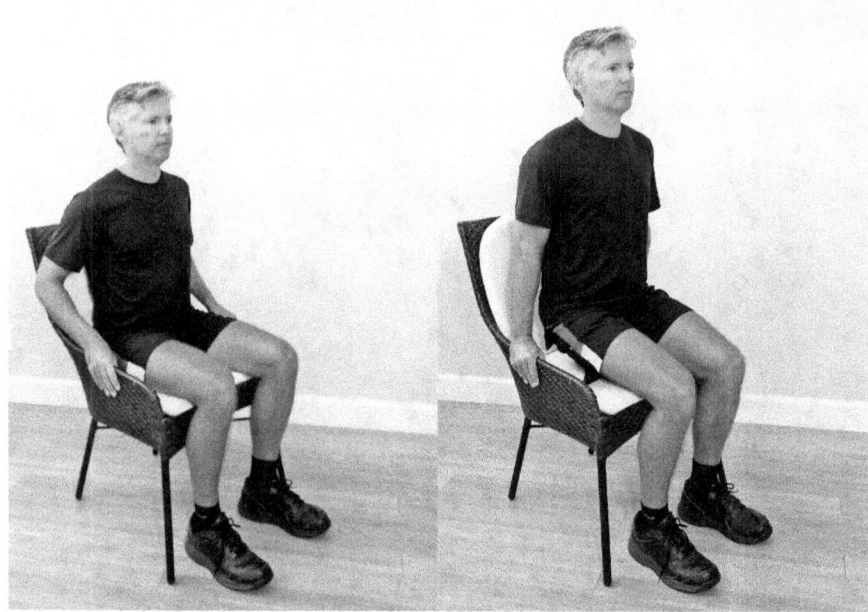

Sit in a sturdy chair with arms. Plant your feet on the floor and grasp the arms. Exhale as you use your arms to lift your body upward. Inhale as you lower your body back into the seat. Repeat 8-12 times.

17. Abdominal Crunches – strengthens stomach muscles.

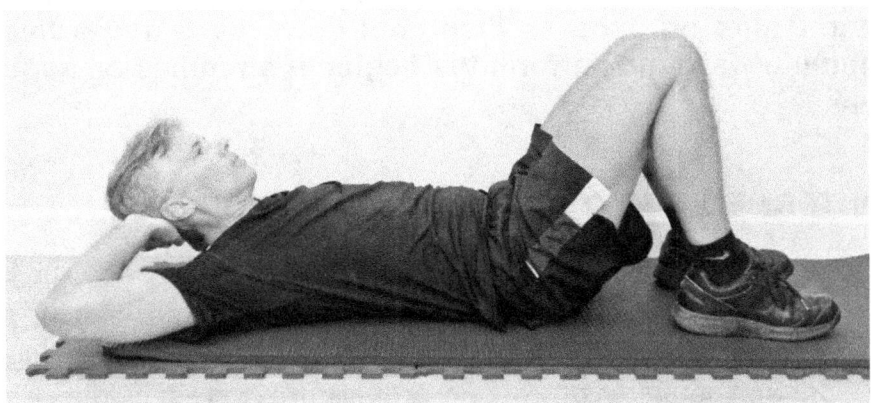

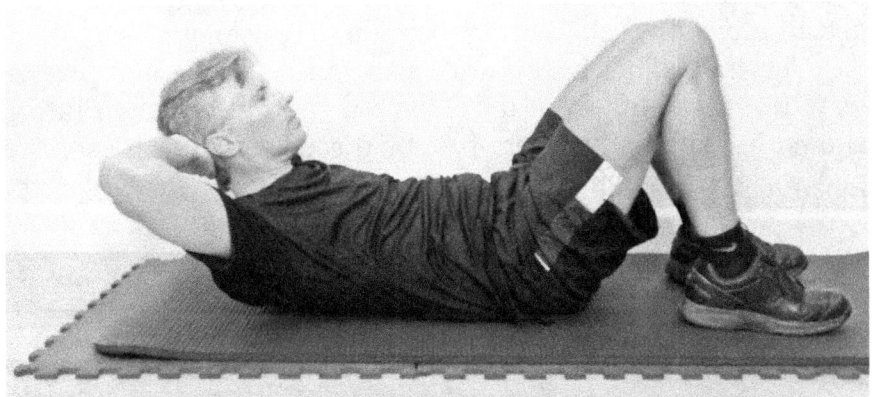

This is for people who are able to get down and up off the floor. Lie down on a mat and bend your knees and plant your feet on the floor. Put your hands behind your head with your elbows flared out. Exhale as you use your abdominal (stomach) muscles to lift your head and shoulders – but not your whole back – as far as you can off the floor. Inhale when you lower to the starting position. Repeat 8-15 times.

COOL DOWN AND STRETCHING

Read about the importance of cooling down and stretching on page 45 then cool down by taking a five minute walk and perform the beginner stretches on page 46.

INTERMEDIATE STRENGTH TRAINING ROUTINE

This exercise routine is for reasonably fit people who have experience working with free weights. When you are retrieving, exercising with, and returning weights, always maintain complete control and proper form to reduce the risk of injury. If you have trouble crouching to lift weights, consider getting a weight rack to bring them up to waist level.

The first panel in this exercise routine shows the proper way to lift weights from the floor. Experienced weight lifters should be able to complete two or three sets of each exercise per workout session.

1. Squat – strengthens upper leg, buttocks, and hips. IMPORTANT NOTE: This is also the proper way to retrieve free weights for your workout, exercising, and returning them.

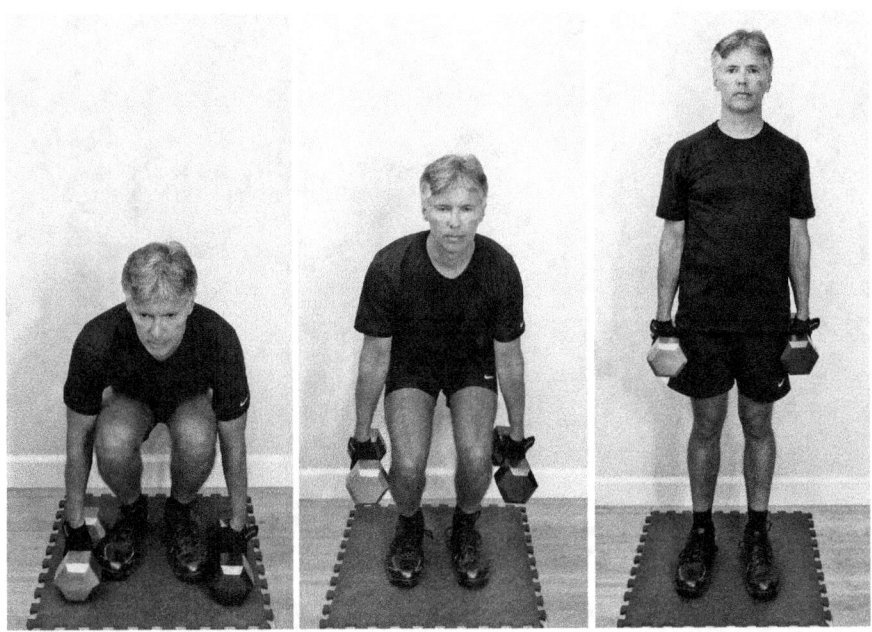

With feet firmly planted on the floor and straight back in line with your neck, inhale as you crouch and grasp the dumbbells with palms aimed in toward your body. Do not allow your knees to extend beyond your toes and do not drop your rear end lower than your knees. Engage your core – abdominal and back muscles – to protect your back and exhale as you slowly rise using your thighs for power. Repeat 10-12 times. Practice this without weights to make sure you have proper form before adding weights.

2. Dumbbell Curl – works the shoulders, front of the upper arm, lower arm, and wrists.

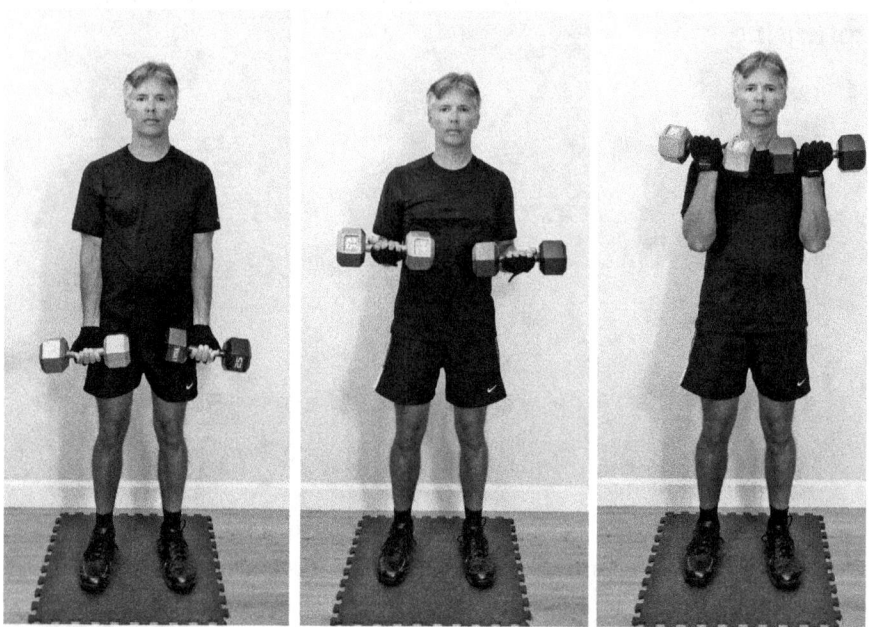

Stand straight, hold the dumbbells with palms forward, slowly exhale as you raise them to shoulder level. Inhale when you return them all the way down to the starting position. Stand with one foot forward if needed for extra balance. Repeat 8-12 times.

3. Triceps Extensions – works the shoulders, back of the upper arms, lower arms, and wrists.

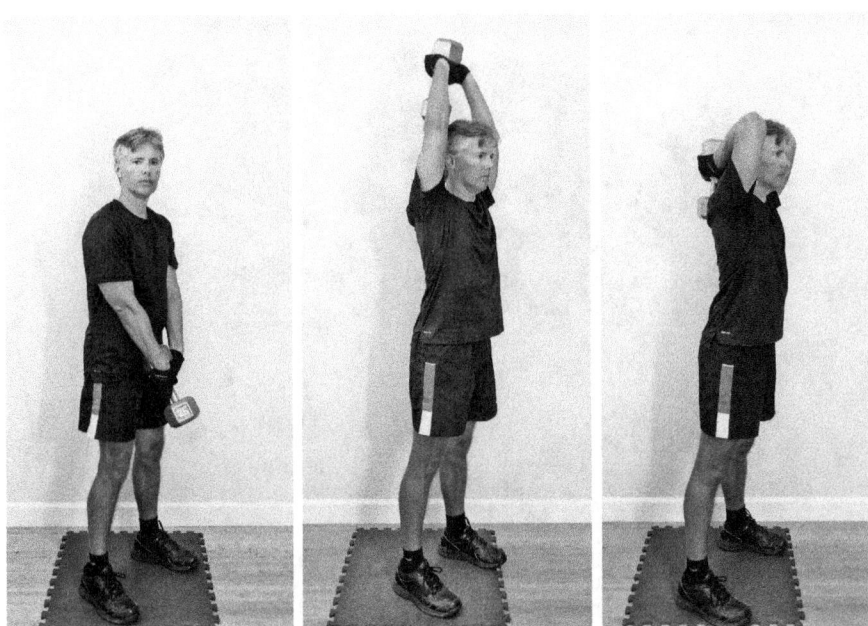

With feet planted shoulder width apart and back straight, hold the end of one dumbbell in both hands. Exhale and raise the dumbbell in front of you and up over the back of your head. Inhale, then exhale as you lower the dumbbell behind your head while keeping your upper arms close to your ears. Exhale as you raise the dumbbell over your head again, inhale, then exhale as you lower it down behind your head again. Keep your abdominal muscles engaged throughout this exercise and don't lock your knees or elbows. Repeat 8-12 times.

4. Push-ups – strengthens chest, shoulders, arms, wrists, and core muscles.

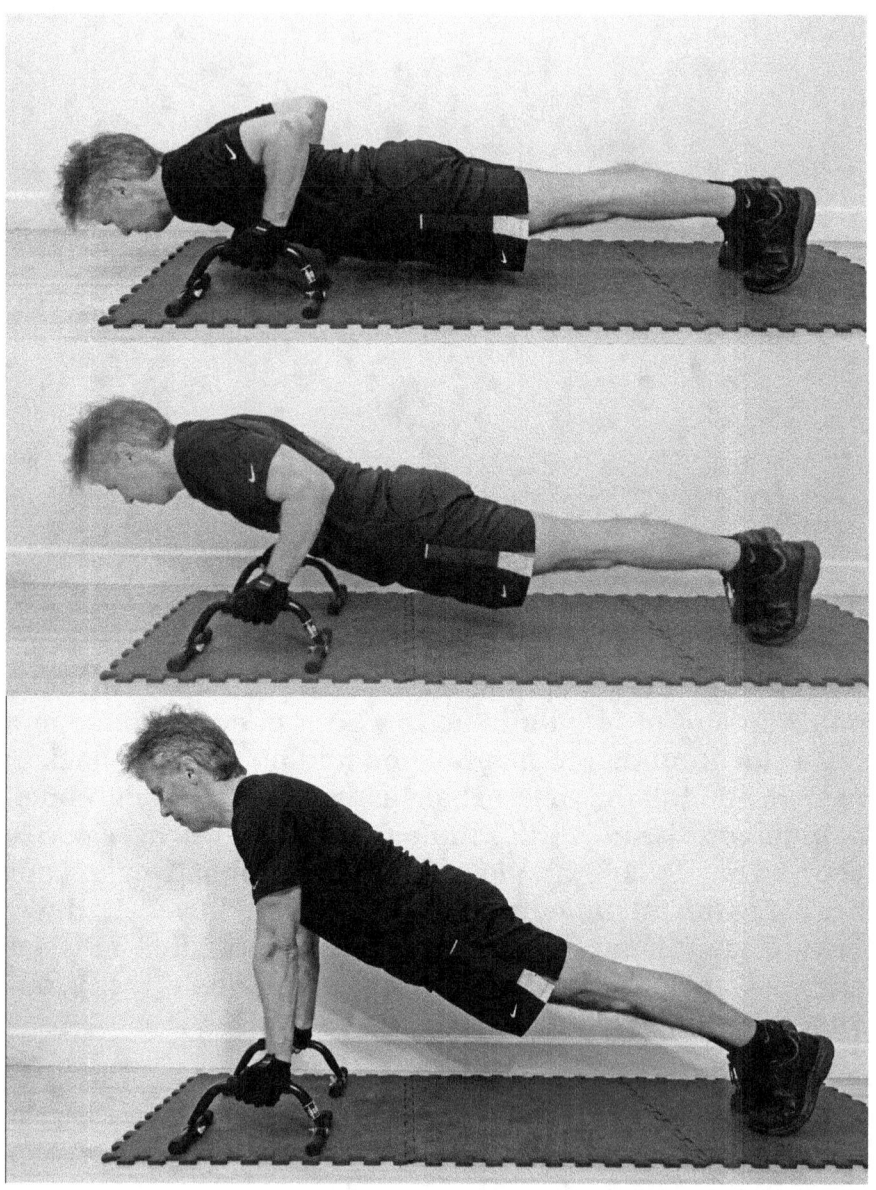

With hands just outside shoulder-width apart grasping push-up bars or palms flat on the floor and feet close together with toes on the floor, engage your abdominal muscles and exhale as you slowly straighten your arms to raise your body off the floor. Keep your head aligned with your straight back and legs. Pause at the top and inhale, then slowly exhale as you lower yourself to the starting position. If push-ups are difficult for you, you can perform modified pushups on your knees. Repeat 8-12 times.

5. Bent Over Rows – works your back and shoulders.

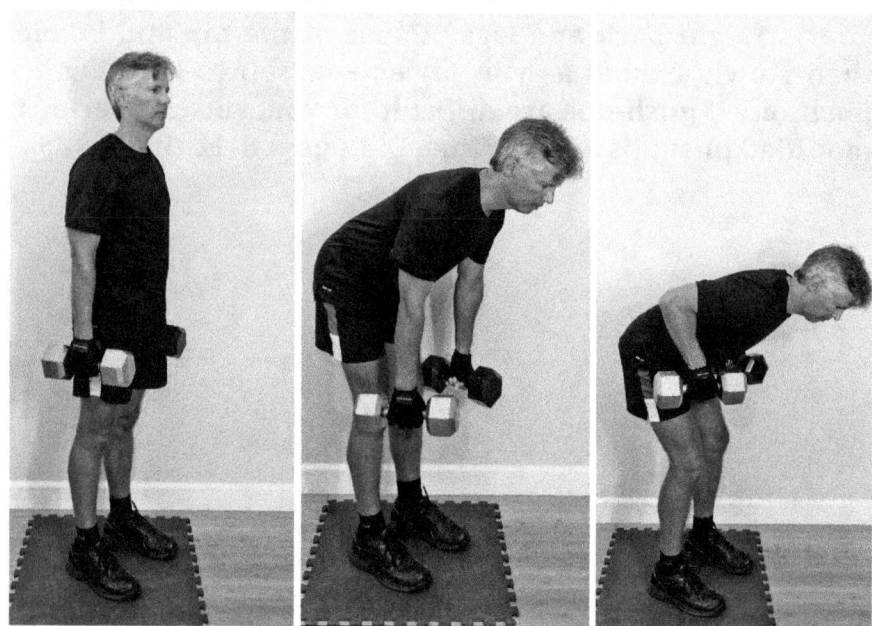

Stand straight holding the dumbbells with your palms in toward your body. With abdominal and back muscles engaged, bend slightly at the knees and exhale as you slowly bend at the waist while keeping your head in line with your back until you reach a 45 degree angle. Inhale. Exhale as you raise the dumbbells back to the height of your stomach, hold, then inhale as you drop them back down. Remain in the bent over position and row the weights 8-12 times. When you're through, exhale as you slowly raise yourself back up to the standing position. Be careful not to arch your back during this exercise. If you feel a tweak in your lower back, check your form, use less weight, or find a substitute exercise that works the same muscles.

6. Squat, Hammer, Shoulder Press – this compound exercise works thighs, arms, and shoulders. Basically three exercises in one, It must be performed with total control and proper form to avoid injury.

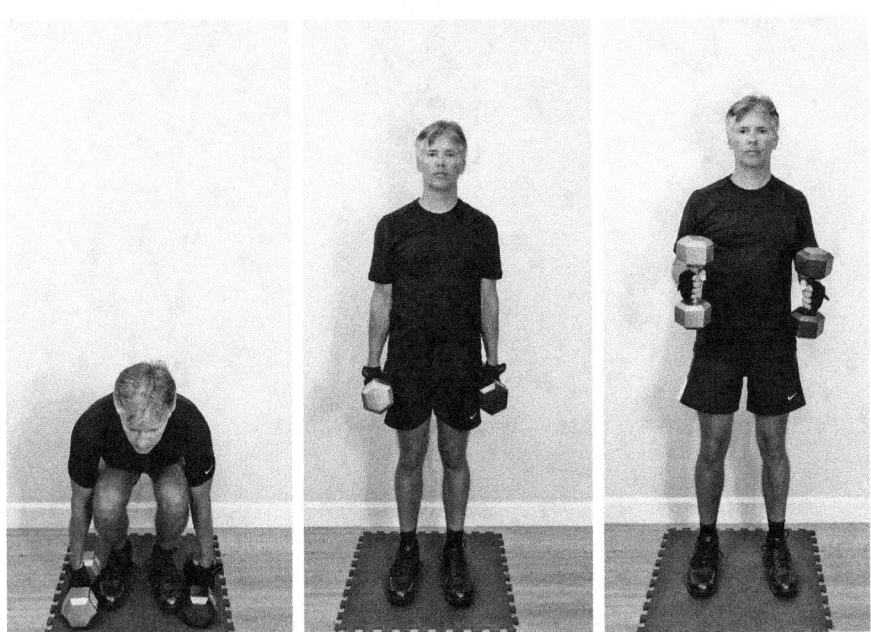

Squat: With feet firmly planted on the ground and straight back in line with your neck, inhale as you crouch and grasp the dumbbells with palms aimed in toward your body. Do not allow your knees to extend beyond your toes and do not drop your rear end lower than your knees. Engage your abdominal and back muscles to protect your back and exhale as you slowly rise using your thighs for power. Practice this without weight to make sure you have proper form before using weight.

Hammer: Stand straight with palms facing in toward your body. Do not lock your knees. Exhale as you slowly hammer curl the weights up to your shoulders.

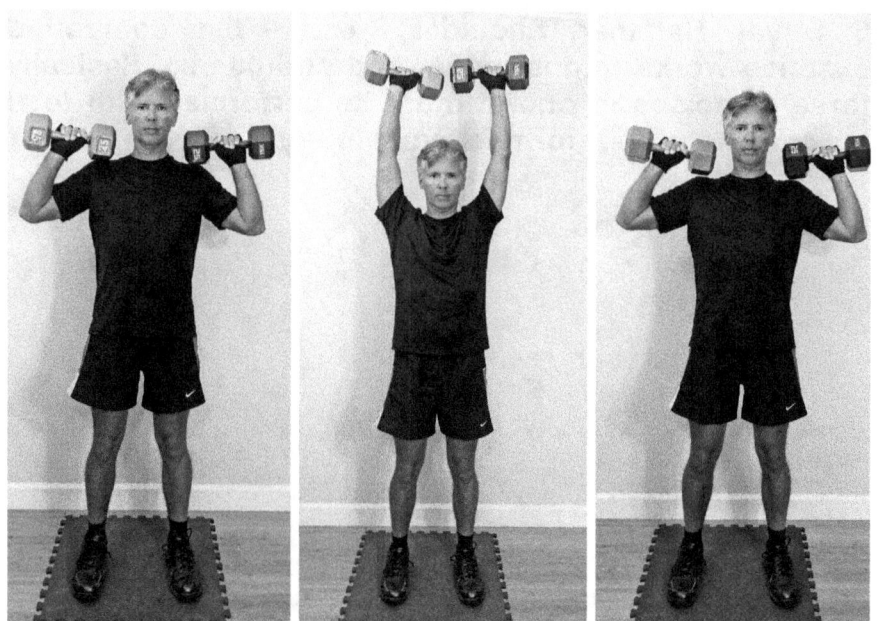

Shoulder Press: With the weights just above your shoulders, turn them to the palm-forward position and inhale. Exhale as you raise the weights straight above your head. Hold for a second and inhale. Exhale as you lower the weights back down to just above your shoulders. Inhale and turn the palms back in toward your body.

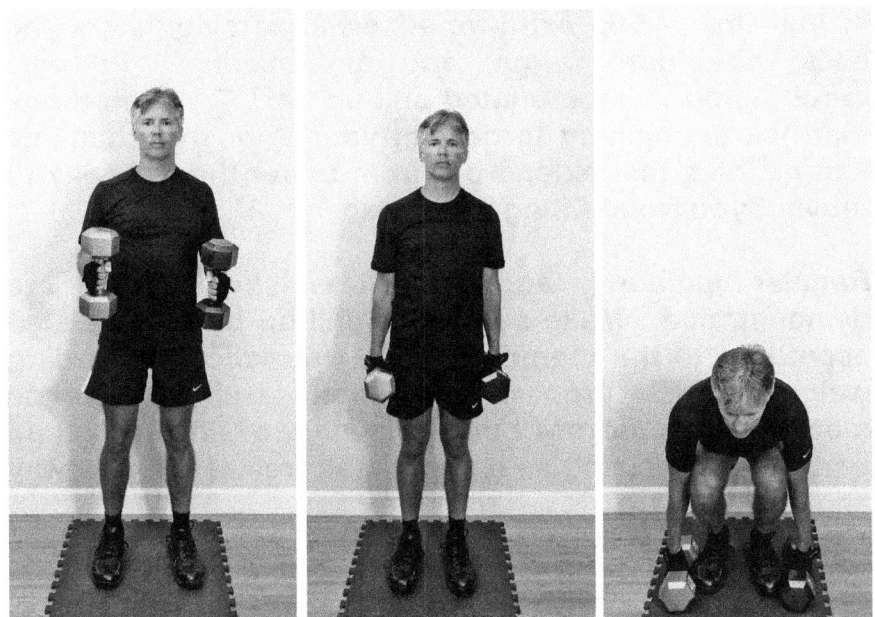

Exhale as you slowly hammer the weights down to your hips. Inhale, then exhale as you squat back down to the starting position. Repeat 8-12 times. This must be performed with total control and proper form to get the most strength training benefit without injury. Practice the move without weights until you feel you can comfortably execute it with weights.

7. Pull-Ups – this extra-for-experts exercise works the back, shoulders, arms, and abdominals. Pull-ups require a doorway mounted pull-up bar. Try to find one that has cushioning to protect your door from damage and handles that extend out from under the doorway to prevent you from hitting your head.

Regular pull-ups and chair assist pull-ups are demonstrated. Make sure your pull-up bar is operated according to the manufacturer's instructions regarding weight limits, proper installation, and appropriate motion. Also, do not bounce, swing, or lift the pull-up bar while exercising as it may break free of the doorway and lead to injury.

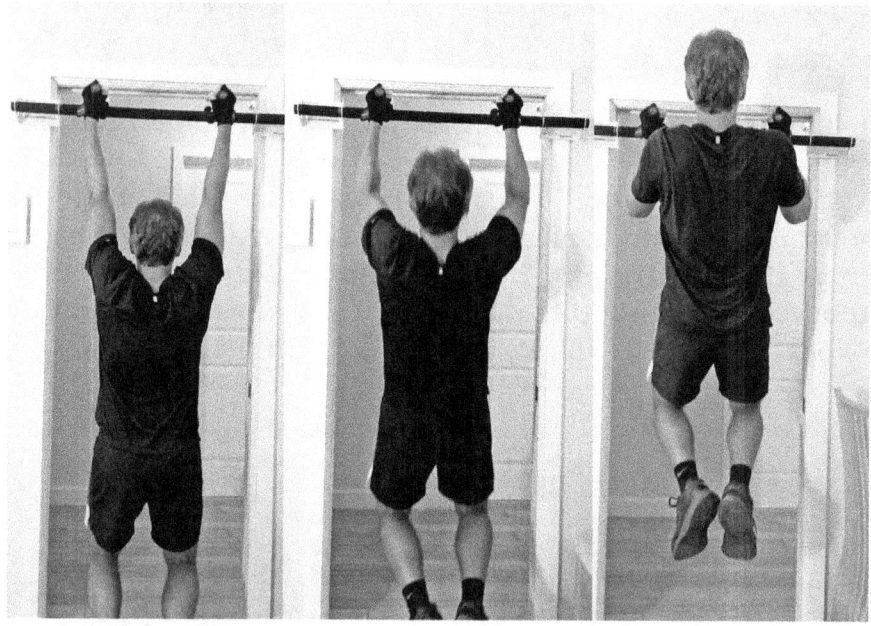

Regular Pull-ups: stand beneath the pull-up bar, grasp the handles and pull downward to make sure the bar is installed correctly. If it is, lower your body at the knees until your arms are straight and holding the load of your body. Exhale as you pull your body up to the point where your chin is just above the bar. Hold for a second. Inhale as you lower your body to the starting position. Keep your back straight and your knees beneath your body throughout the movement. Go slowly and, again, do not swing, bounce, or lift the bar. Repeat 8-12 times.

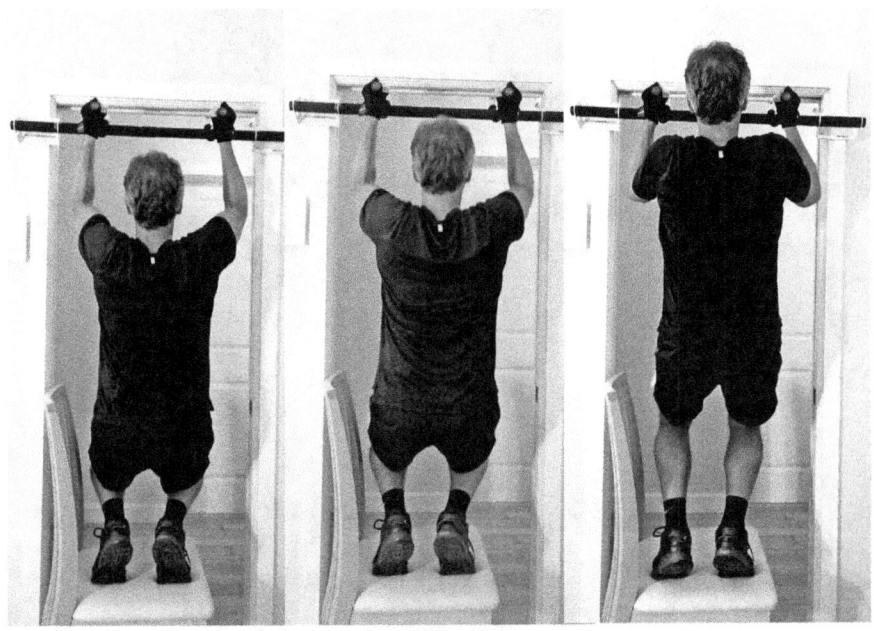

Chair Assist Pull-Ups: Perform this exercise if you are unable to do regular pull-ups. You should have someone spot for you. Place a sturdy chair under the pull-up bar. Stand on the chair and grasp the handles. Crouch down. Primarily use your arms to pull your body upward, but also engage your legs if you need the assist. Do not lift the bar, pull or push the bar, or bounce or swing on it. Repeat 8-12 times, stop in a standing position, release the handles and carefully get down off the of the chair. Perform this version of pull-ups until you gain enough strength to execute pull-ups without assistance from your legs.

8. Crunches – strengthens abdominal muscles.

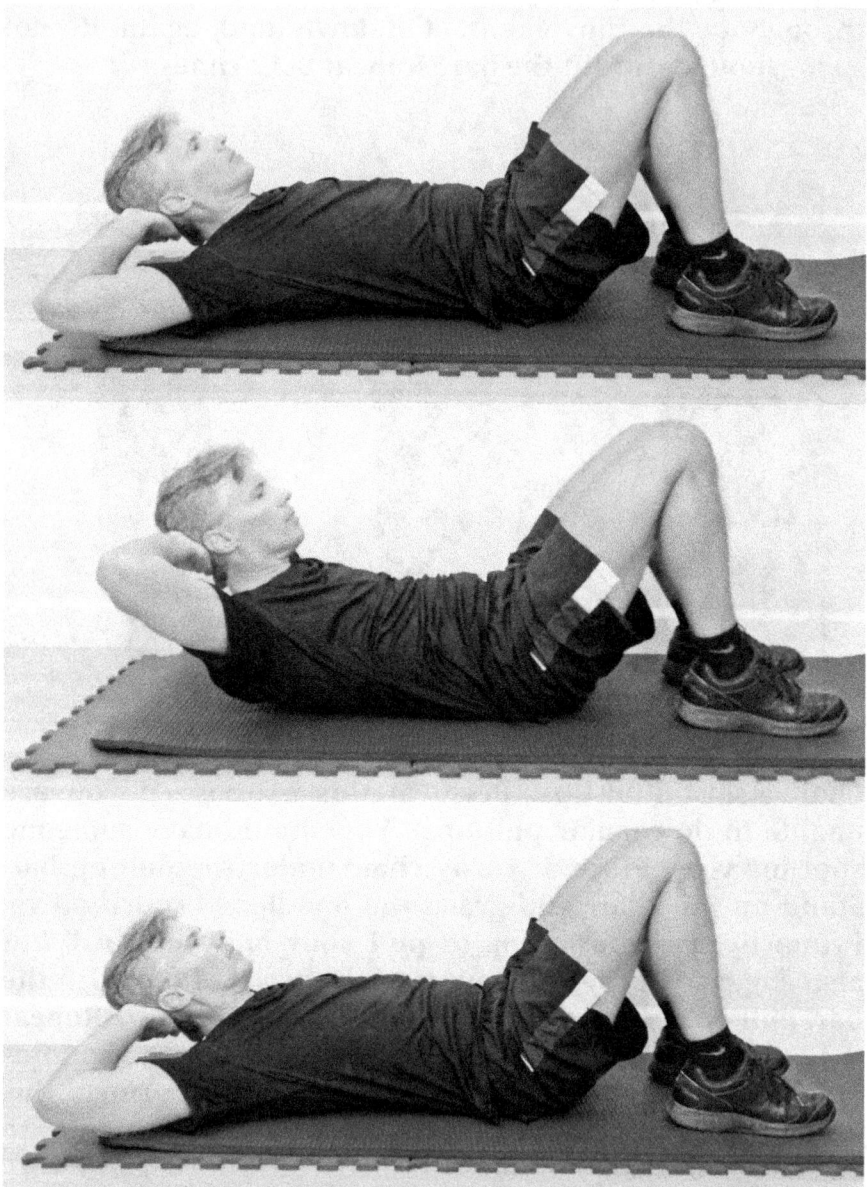

Lie down on a mat and bend your knees and plant your feet on the floor. Put your hands behind your head with your elbows beside your head. Exhale as you use your abdominal muscles to lift your shoulders as far as you can

off the floor.   Inhale when you lower to the starting position. Repeat 8-15 times.

9. Torso Twists – strengthens side abdominal muscles and hips.

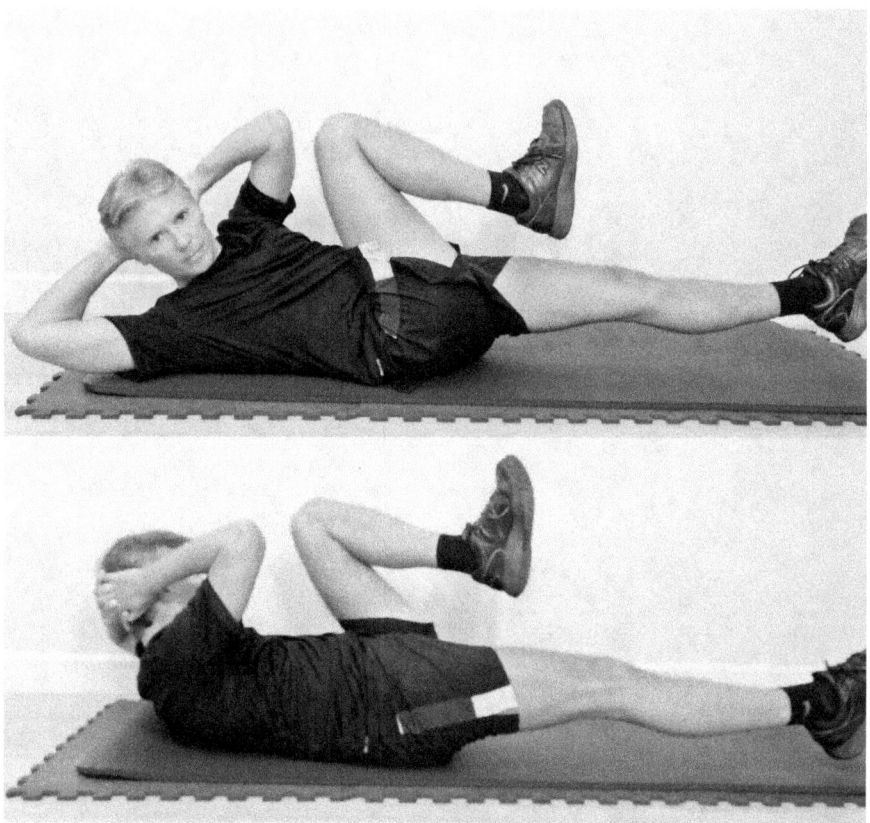

Lie on the mat and place your hands behind your head. Lift both legs an inch or two off the ground, and slowly bring your right elbow to your left knee and then your left elbow to your right knee. Do not lift your back, only your shoulders and legs. Perform the exercise in smooth, rhythmic fashion and remember to breathe. If you can't touch your shoulder to your knee, get as close as you can. Each right knee and left knee tap is one repetition. Complete 8-15 repetitions per leg.

COOL DOWN AND STRETCHING

Read about the importance of cooling down and stretching on page 45 then cool down by taking a five minute walk and perform the intermediate stretches on page 53.

FINAL THOUGHTS

A small investment in strength training – two or three 30-45 minute sessions a week – will have an enormous positive impact on our health as we age. Exercising with resistance gives us the strength we need to go about our everyday activities and the mobility we need to explore and engage our world. Most people want independence as they age. Strength training plays a critical role in achieving that dream.

Fortunately, with so many strength training options, finding a method that works for you shouldn't be too hard. Portable exercise equipment, like resistance bands, make it impossible to miss an exercise session even when you're on the road. Take the time to explore and participate in strength training and be patient as you're building strength and you'll be amazed at what you can accomplish.

Now let's take a look at the fourth pillar in our plan to age well: Eating healthy.

Lawrence S. Richardson, Jr.

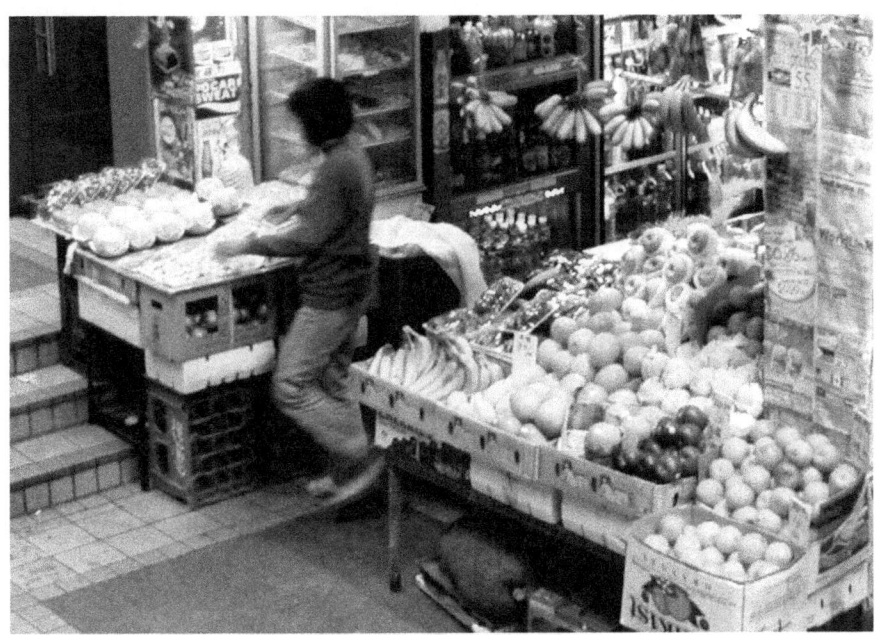

5 HEALTHY DIET ESSENTIALS

Dieting Recommendations:

> **Active women need about 2,000 calories a day. Active men need about 2,400 calories a day.**

> **The diet should be rich in fresh fruits and vegetables, whole grains, non-fat dairy, lean meat and fish in small portions, beans, legumes and nuts.**

> **The diet should avoid heavily processed foods that are loaded with empty calories and fat, oil, sugar, and salt.**

> **Eat only when you are truly hungry**

All the exercise in the world won't improve your weight or general health if you eat a poor diet. **In fact, researchers are convinced a healthy diet is more important than exercise**

for actual weight loss, though exercise will help you keep the weight off and ensure your body is fit.

Believe it or not, there are actually people who are thin but unhealthy because they eat poorly or don't give their bodies the exercise they need to promote a healthy heart and lungs and the strength and balance they need for everyday activities. The bottom line is: Everything you eat and drink is absorbed into your body and impacts how it performs.

A diet that's rich in natural foods – fresh fruits, vegetables, whole grains, non-fat dairy, lean meat and fish, and beans, legumes and nuts – will provide the fuel you need to power through your day. A diet that's loaded with heavily processed foods that are full of empty calories and fat, oil, sugar, and salt will make you sluggish and cause you to pile on the pounds.

Transitioning from an unhealthy diet to a healthy diet and staying there isn't easy. If it were, two-thirds of Americans wouldn't be obese or overweight. Part of the problem is the overabundance of high-calorie, low-nutrition food readily available at countless restaurants, convenience stores and grocery stores. It's almost impossible to escape it, but you must if you want to be fitter and age well.

ASK YOUR PHYSICIAN FOR DIETING ADVICE

Your doctor is a valuable resource for credible dieting advice. Unfortunately, many doctors do not initiate weight-related discussions for fear of offending their patients. That means it's up to you to bring up the subject. Speaking with your doctor is important because he or she can:

1. Provide dieting advice based on your specific physical condition and health challenges, such as heart disease or diabetes.

2. Tell you more precisely the number of calories you should consume each day to maintain a healthy weight or to lose weight based on your size, age, and activity level.

3. Help you to set realistic, achievable goals.

4. Monitor your progress.

5. Refer you to a registered dietitian.

CONSIDER WORKING WITH A DIETICIAN

A registered dietician, either on an individual basis or in a credible group program, such as Weight Watchers, can:

1. Provide you with more intensive attention than your doctor.

2. Provide you with realistic, effective strategies to eat healthier that are tailored to your lifestyle and tastes.

3. Monitor your progress and reward you for major accomplishments.

4. Motivate you to adopt healthier eating habits and stick with them.

5. Invite you to join a group, which, research has shown, is more effective than dieting alone.

6. Modify your diet, when necessary, to ensure you reach your goals.

When you visit a dietician, insist on a diet that is rich in basic, easily-attainable foods. If he or she pushes expensive nutritional supplements and exotic foods and beverages, or stresses single, silver bullet foods, with the promise that they will solve all your health challenges, find another dietician.

TRY THE NON-DIET DIET

Those who want to take a less-intensive approach to dieting might want to try the Non-diet Diet. This involves changing your habits by taking pro-active steps to build a healthy diet by reducing or eliminating unhealthy foods.

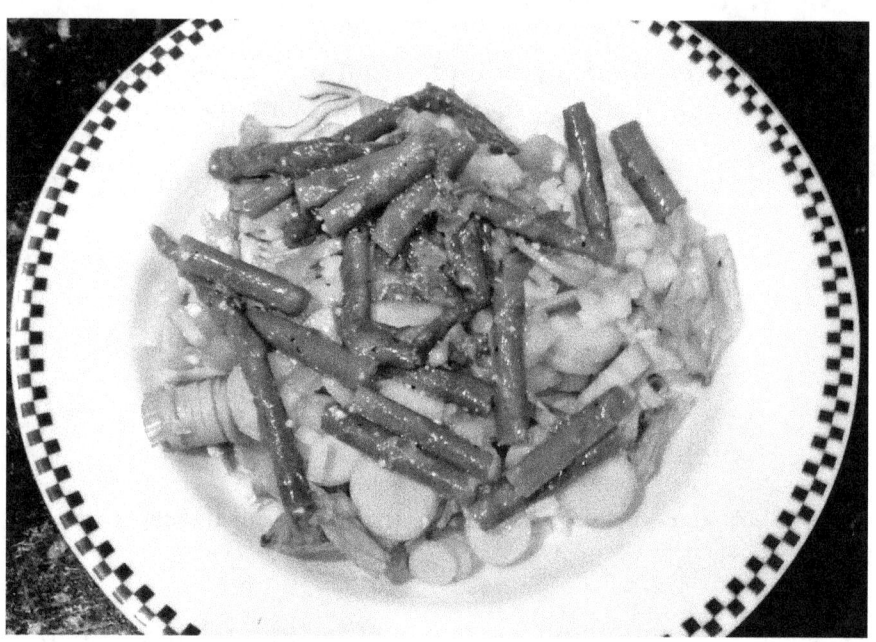

What Is A Healthy Diet?

You can't build a healthy diet if you don't know what one is. A healthy diet is consuming your recommended number of calories a day, or less if you're trying to lose weight, and building a menu that:

➢ Is rich in fresh vegetables and fruits.

➢ Substitutes whole grain rice, pastas, breads, and cereals for potatoes and heavily processed starches like white bread, white rice, and regular pastas.

➢ Restricts red meat consumption – if any at all – to a few

servings a week.

➢ Delivers protein through healthy boneless, skinless white meat chicken, fish, non-fat dairy products, and nuts, beans, and other legumes.

A healthy diet eliminates or minimizes:

➢ Processed foods, which are usually loaded with unhealthy fat, oil, sugar, and salt.

➢ Sugary sodas, juices – even fruit juices, which lack fiber – and supposedly healthy sports drinks.

➢ Coffee and other beverages made with cream and sugar.

➢ Fatty meats, such as marbled steak and skin-on or dark meat chicken and turkey.

➢ High fat dairy products, including whole milk, cream, and cheese.

➢ Fried foods, such as French fries, fried chicken, and potato chips.

➢ Snacks full of empty calories, such as ice cream, candy, cookies, and cake.

➢ Supposedly natural or organic foods that are full of empty calories, sugar, and salt.

The last point comes as a surprise to many people. Not all foods that are labeled natural or organic are good for you. For example, many granola cereals contain excessive amounts of raw sugar, which is the same as refined sugar to your body. And potato chips that contain natural sea salt are no better for you than chips that are coated in regular salt. They're both fried in oil and have high amounts of sodium.

With empty calories, oil, fat, sugar, and salt routinely hidden in processed foods, it's more important than ever to take a look at ingredients and nutritional value labels regardless of the health benefit the manufacturer is hyping on the front of the box.

15 QUICK DIETING TIPS

Just like any diet, the Non-Diet Diet calls on people to change their behaviors. Here are a few tips to help you on your way:

1. **Keep processed and other unhealthy foods out of your home.** Out of sight, out of mind is true. Studies have shown people tend to eat a poor diet when unhealthy food is convenient. Don't let unhealthy and heavily processed foods into your house or workplace and you will be less likely to eat them.

2. **Fill your refrigerator and cupboard with healthy foods.** If you have easy access to healthy foods, like fresh fruit and vegetables, whole wheat bread, non-fat dairy products – like yogurt – and nuts (which should be eaten in moderation) – you will eat a healthier diet.

3. **Eat three meals a day.** Eating three meals a day and a few healthy snacks in between when you are truly hungry – not just out of habit or boredom – will keep you from swinging between starvation and binge eating calorie-laden foods.

4. **Avoid excessive snacking.** When it comes to unwanted weight gain, it's the little numbers that get you. If you must snack, substitute fat free yogurt for ice cream, low calorie granola bars for candy bars and baked goods, and fruit for sugary drinks, including fresh juices with the fiber removed..

5. **Eat out only as an occasional treat.** When eating out, it's nearly impossible to limit oil, fat, sugar, and salt. Instead, save eating at a restaurant or ordering take-out food for special occasions. Enjoy the treat then return to your healthy diet.

6. **Let others have the leftovers.** When you do eat out, have the server wrap up the leftovers and give the doggy bag to someone else. More than one meal of calorie-laden restaurant food is damaging and can lead you to break your healthy diet.

7. **Prepare your meals at home.** Preparing meals at home is best because you can be assured that the ingredients are fresh and free of harmful ingredients. It's also keeps you on your feet, which is good for your overall health.

8. **Sneak vegetables into all your dishes.** You can fill yourself up with healthy vegetables by sneaking them into dishes from omelets to meatloaf. Find out how in the recipe section at the end of this chapter.

9. **Prepare your plate before you sit down at the table.** Divide your meal into a quarter healthy meat or fish, a quarter whole grains, just over a quarter vegetables, and just under a quarter fruit, and you'll be on the road to good health.

10. **Eat a healthy meal before you go to a party.** Arriving at a party satisfied, will cut down on your craving for the unhealthy fare served at most parties. Also, when you get there, load up on salad and cut vegetables and skip any dishes involving chips, heavy dips, cheese, unhealthy meats, and deserts.

11. **Don't stand in the kitchen or near the buffet table.** Standing near food at a party inevitably leads to talking

and habitual binge eating.

12. **Remember alcohol packs a lot of empty calories.**
Wine, beer, and a shot of spirits can range anywhere
from 100 to 150 calories each per drink, which can
really add up. Decide how much you are going to drink
at a party – if at all – before you go and stick to the limit.

13. **Put notes on your refrigerator and cupboard.** Casual
snacking is a tough habit to break. To snap out of the
trance of habitual eating, stick notes on your
refrigerator and cupboard doors that remind you of
your health goals. The message can be as simple as "Are
you really hungry?" or "Why not go for a walk instead?"

14. **Drink water with every meal.** Drinking water with
every meal builds volume and a sense of fullness. It also
aids in digestion.

15. **Don't watch food TV or read foodie magazines.**
Frequent exposure to the foods featured on these
programs that are usually rich in meat, cheese, fat, and
oil will make you crave them. Restrict your media food
diet to programs that promote healthy foods.

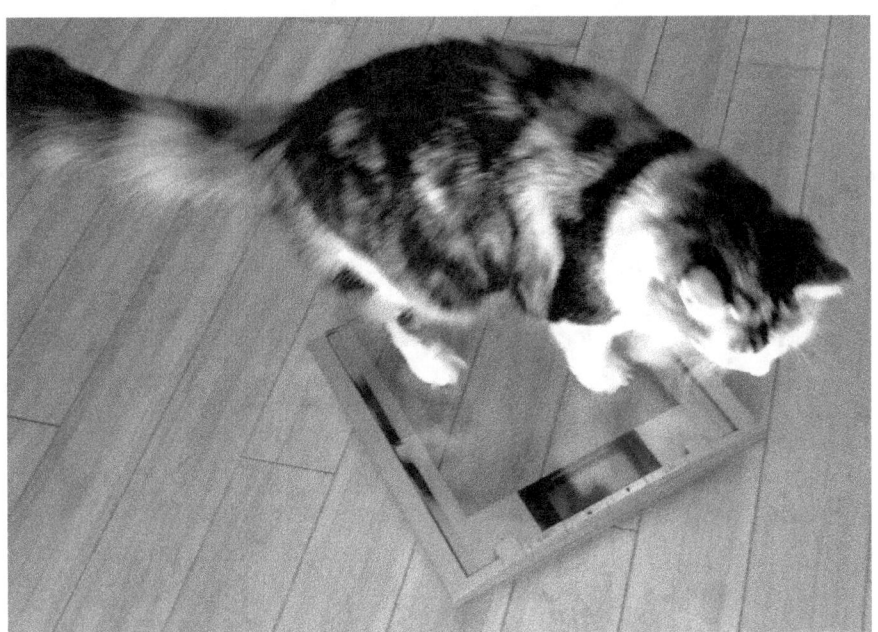

Measure Your Starting Point And Your Progress

One valuable tool to determine whether or not losing weight should be one of your fitness goals is measuring your Body Mass Index (BMI) using a BMI calculator. You can find a BMI calculator by going to Google.com and entering in the search terms "BMI Calculator." The first resource should be the National Heart Lung and Blood Institute's link.

Go to the site's BMI Calculator, enter your height and weight, and the calculator will give you your BMI. It will also tell you if you are underweight, just right, or overweight. Beware, however, that BMI does not give an accurate reading for people who have certain characteristics, such as being very muscular or short. If you are, you might need to consult your doctor for a more accurate take.

To establish your benchmark weight and track your progress, it's important to weigh yourself at the same time and under the same circumstances once a week. Why? Because your weight varies throughout the day – due to factors such as eating meals and the loss of water weight from aerobic exercise. The best time to weigh yourself is when you first wake up – but not the morning after you ate an unusually large meal or drank a lot of alcoholic beverages – since no other factors will skew your weight. Also, don't rely on your memory. Write the number down in a journal to make sure you're headed in the right direction.

One final point, if you're working out heavily with weights, the weight gain you see just might be muscle weight, which is a good thing.

10 FREQUENTLY ASKED QUESTIONS

1. **What is the most effective way to lose weight?** Unless your physician prescribes weight loss medicine or stomach banding, a healthy diet with less calories than you burn in a day combined with exercise is the most effective long-term weight-loss strategy.

2. **What's the best way to lose belly or hip weight?** There is no way to target weight loss. When you diet, your body will lose weight across the board.

3. **How should I begin eating a healthier diet?** A great place to start is by taking a look in your refrigerator and cupboard and seeing if you're eating a lot of processed foods that are laden with empty calories, oil, fat, sugar, and salt. If they're there, chances are you're eating them. Eliminating them from your home and replacing them with healthy foods is a great place to start transitioning to a health diet.

4. **Should I take vitamins and other nutritional supplements?** You should only take vitamins and other nutritional supplements with your doctor's approval. Health researchers are increasingly finding that people who take vitamins and other nutritional supplements, such as fish oil with omega 3, may actually be more

prone to disease. Additionally, Congress passed a law that prevents the U.S. Food & Drug Administration from policing manufacturers of vitamins and nutritional supplements the way they regulate the prescription drug industry, so there is no way to be sure you're getting a quality product that delivers real health benefits. In other words, unless your doctor prescribes vitamins or nutritional supplements, get the nutrition you need from a healthy diet.

5. **Should I skip meals to lose weight?** No. The problem with skipping meals is it makes you so hungry that you will binge on calorie-laden foods to make up for the deficit when snacking or at your next meal. It's better not to starve yourself, but to eat an appropriate amount of healthy foods that keep you satisfied throughout the day.

6. **What should I do if I'm hungry between meals?** Eat fresh fruit and vegetables, a low-fat granola bar, or a handful of nuts. Over time, you will get better at determining the amount of food you need to get through the day without eating excessive calories.

7. **Can I eat larger meals if I'm working out?** Many athletes fall into the trap of believing that just because they're working out they can eat like a horse or eat whatever they want. The basic laws of health still apply regardless of the amount of exercise you're getting. You need to consume roughly as many calories as you burn to maintain a health weight and less calories to lose weight.

8. **Do I need to count calories?** If you eat a generally healthy diet and you're satisfied with your weight, no. If you're trying to lose weight, it's a good idea to know how many calories are in the foods you eat. You don't have to be obsessive. Just consider that if you're eating

a thousand calories at breakfast, you just consumed about half of the calories you're allowed in a day. Try to distribute the calories allowed throughout the day to avoid hunger.

9. **What should I do if my partner won't transition to a healthy diet with me?** Whether or not to diet and exercise are very personal health decisions. You can't make someone do either – at least not for very long – if they don't really want to. Therefore, you need to make the commitment yourself. There's always the chance they'll join you when they see your spectacular results. Also, consider joining Weight Watchers or another well-reviewed organization, where you will receive the support you need to reach your goals.

10. **I just cheated and ate a huge meal with desert at a restaurant, what should I do?** Treating yourself occasionally is not the end of the world. Enjoy treats without guilt then get back to your healthy diet.

Losing Weight Requires Patience

You didn't gain excess weight in a day, don't expect to lose it in a day, week, or month. The sensible and gradual approach to weight loss using healthy techniques you can live with is much better for you than using fad diets or medicine not approved by your physician.

HEALTHY RECIPES AND FOOD HANDLING TIPS

A healthy diet doesn't mean going without your favorite, flavorful foods, it means cooking them at home and modifying recipes to remove harmful fat, oil, sugar, and salt. Often, you will discover the dishes you enjoyed at restaurants didn't really need empty calories to begin with, especially if you think of ways to make them delicious by adding tons of vegetables and spices to them.

Following are some recipes to give you an idea of what's possible using a healthier approach to cooking. *(Free printable copies of the recipes and cooking videos are available by entering "recipe" in the search window on Xeniors.com.)* Before you begin cooking, remember to practice safe food handling techniques, such as:

➢ Keep ingredients refrigerated until you're ready to cook.

➢ Don't use the same cutting board or knife to cut meat and vegetables.

➢ Wash your hands thoroughly with soap and hot water before cooking and after handling meats – or wear disposable gloves.

➢ Don't wipe spills off your counter with the same cloth you use to dry your hands.

➢ Wash all surfaces, pans, and utensils with hot soapy water.

➢ Break meals down into smaller portions and put them in your refrigerator to cool them down faster.

➢ Make sure meats are thoroughly cooked.

Follow these tips and you will reduce the risk of food-borne illnesses.

LET'S COOK!

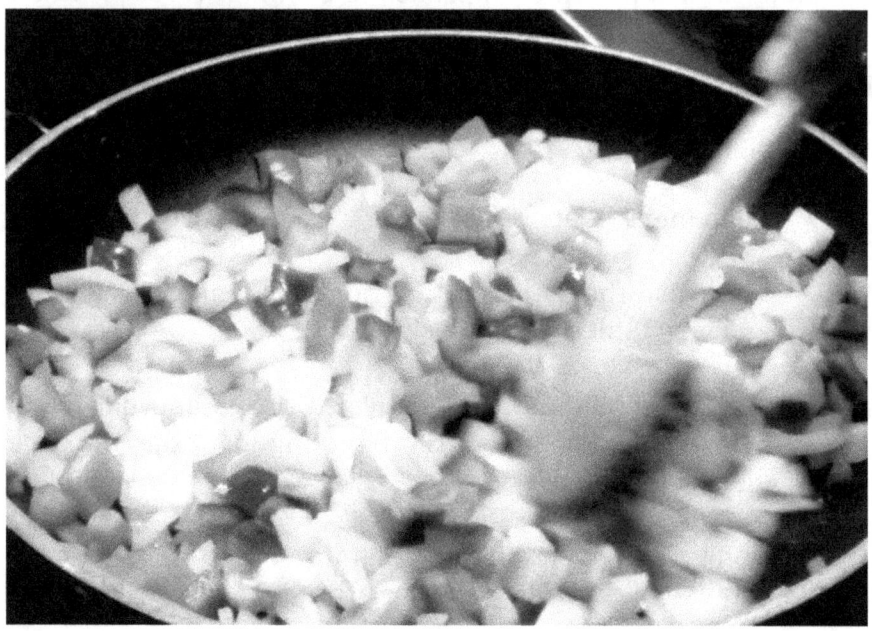

CHICKEN CACCIATORE

This recipe makes traditional chicken cacciatore with boneless, skinless chicken, which means it's low fat and much healthier.

Ingredients:

2 chicken breasts with skin and bone (they will be removed after baking)

1   large box white mushrooms

1   large sweet onion

1   large green pepper

1   head garlic

1/2 teaspoon dried Italian seasonings

6   tablespoons olive oil

2   large cans crushed tomatoes

1   bag yolk-free egg noodles

Instructions:

Preheat oven to 350 degrees. Crush four cloves garlic and combine with 3 tablespoons of olive oil. Insert mix UNDER chicken skin — the skin will be removed after baking. Place chicken on foil and bake for 35 minutes — the chicken will cook more in the simmering cacciatore sauce.

Chop onion and pepper into 1/4 inch chunks. Slice mushrooms into 1/8 inch thick pieces. Place in pan with 3 tablespoons of olive oil and sauté over medium heat for fifteen minutes or until onions begin to turn translucent. Do not brown.

Add vegetables, 1/2 teaspoon of Italian seasonings to large pan containing crushed tomatoes. Simmer over 1/4 heat with lid on pan to prevent spattering. Optional: Add remaining whole cloves of garlic.

Remove chicken from oven. Take off skin and discard. Chop chicken into large 1/2 inch chunks. Pick bones clean and discard bones. Add chicken to the sauce and simmer for 1/2 hour, stirring every 5-10 minutes. Do not overcook sauce.

Serve over egg noodles prepared according to recipe on bag.

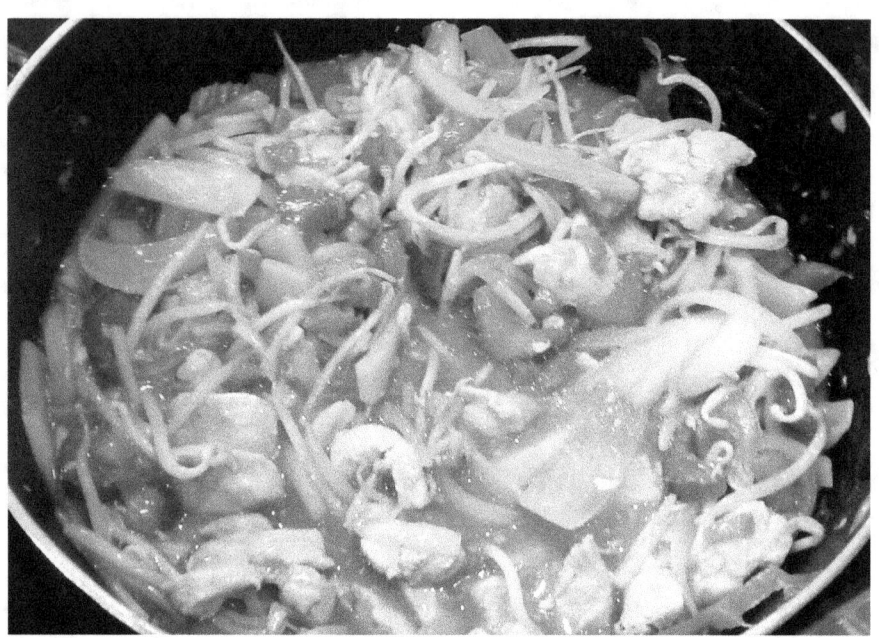

CHICKEN CHOW MEIN

Everyone loves Chinese food. Unfortunately, most restaurant-made Chinese food is extremely high in fat, oil, and sodium. Fortunately, you can make Chinese food at home with boneless, skinless chicken and a fraction of the oil and salt found in the restaurant version and still create a delicious meal.

Ingredients:

2   boneless breasts of chicken

1   bag bean sprouts

3   celery stalks

1   medium onion

1/4 sweet red pepper

1/2 head of garlic

1   can bamboo shoots (optional)

1   red chili pepper

1   can low sodium chicken broth (homemade is even better)

4   tablespoons corn starch

4   tablespoons soy sauce (less, if you prefer)

1   teaspoon Chinese 5 Spices

1/4 teaspoon white pepper

4   servings of rice

Instructions:

Cut the chicken breasts into cubes. Add 1 tablespoon of canola oil to frying pan. Preheat over medium heat. Add chicken pieces and brown until cooked through. Make sure there is no pink visible in the chicken.

Slice the celery stalks into 1/8 of an inch thick pieces. Sliver the onion into thin slices. Dice the sweet red pepper and red hot chili pepper into small pieces. Mince the garlic.

Put one tablespoon of canola oil in a large sauce pan, preheat over medium heat and add the vegetables, including the bamboo shoots. Saute the vegetables until the onions just start to appear clear. Then turn the heat down. You want the vegetables sauteed but still crunchy.

Fill a measuring cup 3/4 full with chicken broth. Add two heaping tablespoons of corn starch, one teaspoon of Chinese 5 Spices, 1/4 teaspoon of white pepper and two tablespoons of soy sauce. Mix well with a fork until there are no clumps.

Add the browned chicken to the vegetable mix. Pour the broth mixture into it and stir it in, then add the beansprouts.

If you like more sauce, make it with the remaining chicken broth and some water to bring the measuring cup to 3/4 full and add the same measure of corn starch and soy sauce as before. Do not add more Chinese 5 Spices or white pepper, as they will overpower the dish.

Heat over medium to low heat, stirring occasionally until sauce thickens. Taste and decide if it needs more spice or soy sauce. You can also add plain water if the sauce gets too thick.

Serve over rice or mixed into low mein noodles.

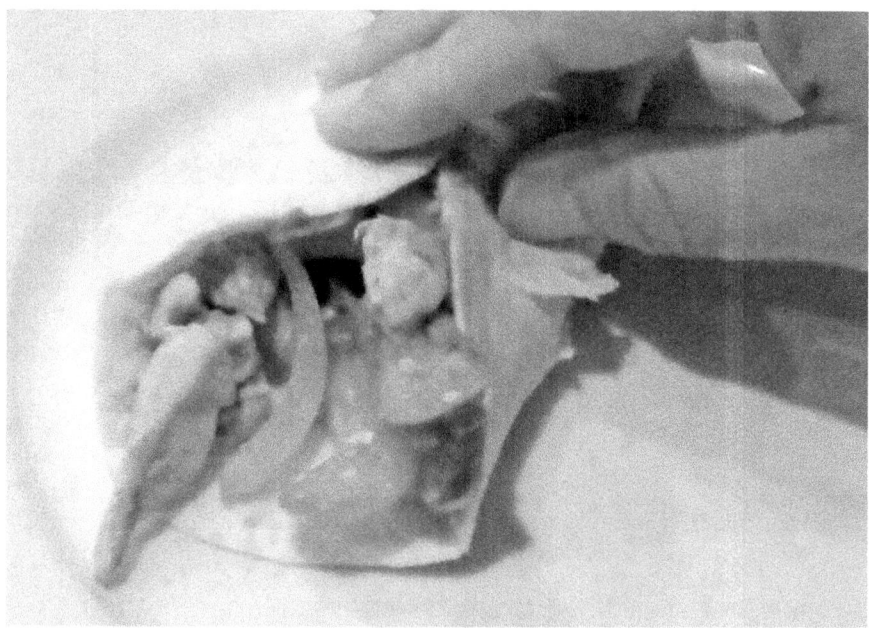

CHICKEN FAJITA BURRITO

The basic chicken fajita burrito consists of a delicious mix of chicken, fresh vegetables, spices, and refried beans rolled up in a flour tortilla. It's an easy, nutritious, and low-fat dish that's sure to be a crowd pleaser.

Ingredients:

2   boneless skinless chicken breasts

1/2 green bell pepper

1/2 red pepper

1   Vidalia onion

1   jalapeno

1/2 teaspoon cumin

1/4 teaspoon salt

1   teaspoon Canola oil

1   can fat-free or vegetarian refried beans

1   pack flour tortillas

Instructions:

Cut the chicken breasts into morsels. Preheat pan over medium heat. Add 1 teaspoon Canola oil, chicken, 1/4 teaspoon cumin, and 1/4 teaspoon salt. Brown chicken.

Sliver the green bell pepper, red pepper, onion, and jalapeno into slivers. When the chicken is browned, put it to the side in the pan, add the vegetables, and saute them until they just start to appear clear.

Warm the refried beans in a sauce pan. Warm a tortilla in a small pan over medium heat. When the tortilla is warmed, but not toasted, remove it from the pan and put some of the chicken and vegetable mix in the tortilla, along with a strip of the refried beans. Now you have a fajita burrito. Serve with baked tortilla chips and salsa.

You can also make this dish with a splash of mojo sauce for added flavor.

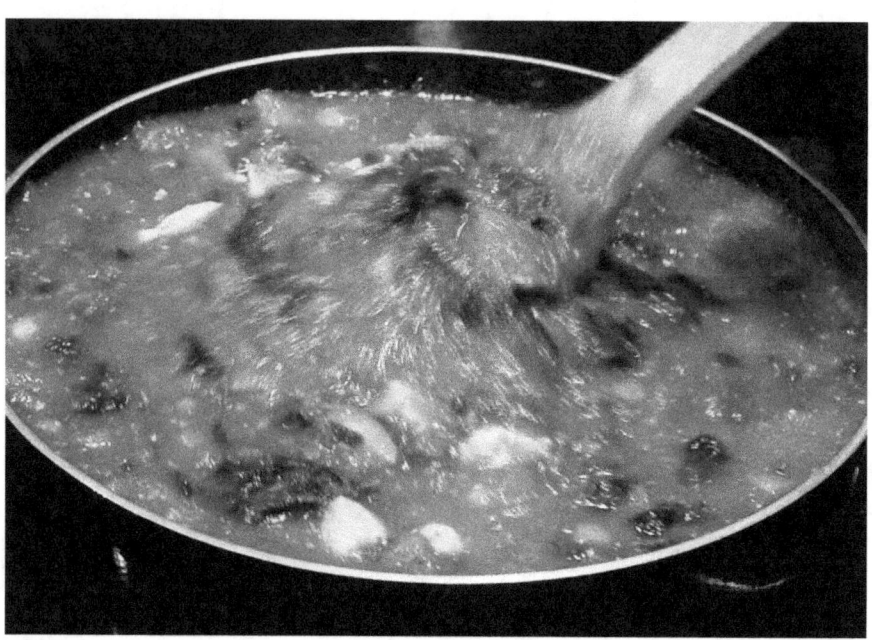

CHICKEN SPINACH VEGETABLE MARINARA

Our healthy Chicken Spinach Vegetable Marinara is absolutely delicious and rich in vegetables with only a tiny amount of fat provided by a few tablespoons of olive oil and boneless, skinless chicken.

Ingredients:

1 1/2 pounds boneless skinless chicken

3   28 ounce cans of crushed tomatoes

2   6 ounce cans of tomato paste

2   bags baby spinach

1   green bell pepper

1   red pepper

1   head garlic

1   large Vidalia onion

2 1/2   tablespoons extra virgin olive oil

1   tablespoon Italian seasonings

1   box multigrain or whole wheat pasta

Instructions:

Pour crushed tomatoes into a large pan and put on 1/4 heat.

Cube the green bell pepper, red pepper, and Vidalia onion and put in a bowl. Crush the garlic on top of the vegetable mix.

Place a frying pan over medium heat, add a tablespoon of olive oil, then pour in the vegetable mix. Saute the vegetables until the onions just start to appear clear. Pour the vegetable mix into the crushed tomatoes and stir in.

Chop the spinach and saute in the frying pan with a tablespoon of olive oil until it's wilted – cooked through. Stir the spinach into the crushed tomatoes and vegetables. If you prefer a vegetarian dish, you can skip the next step – adding browned chicken.

Chop the chicken into half-inch pieces and brown in the frying pan with a teaspoon of olive oil. When no pink is showing, add the chicken to the marinara mix.

Stir a tablespoon of Italian seasoning into the marinara. If you prefer your marinara on the thick side, stir in one or two cans of tomato paste.

Allow the marinara to simmer over low heat for a half hour, stirring occasionally, then serve over multigrain or wheat pasta.

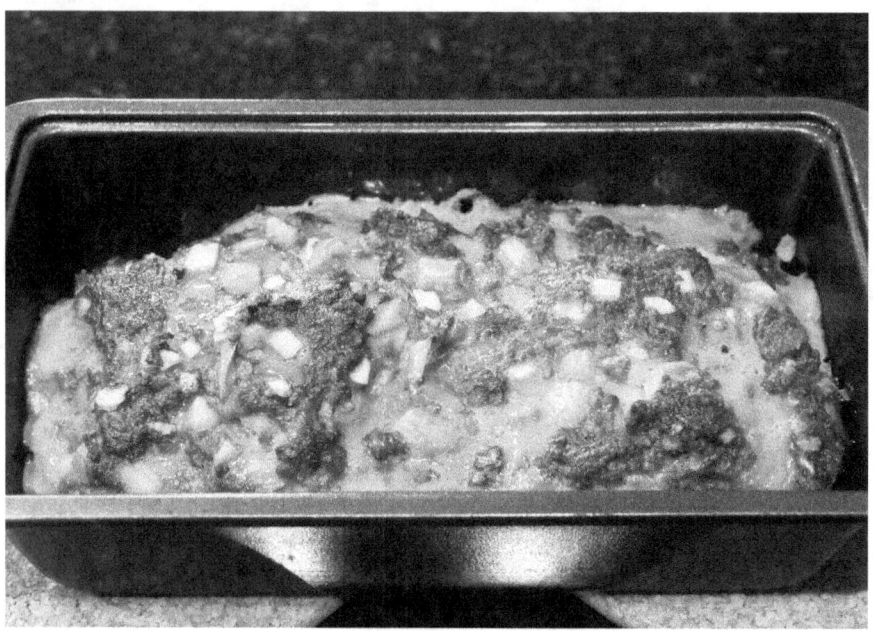

MEATLOAF

Even a dish as meaty as meatloaf can be made healthier and tastier with a healthy dose of vegetables.

Ingredients:

2 lbs	lean hamburger
2	pieces toasted whole wheat bread
1	onion (3/4 cups chopped)
1	green or red pepper (3/4 cups chopped)
2	eggs

4	cloves garlic
1	teaspoon Italian seasoning mix
1	teaspoon black pepper
	Canola oil non-stick spray

Instructions:

Preheat your oven to 375 degrees.

Take the toasted bread and either chop it up into tiny pieces or run it through your food processor to make breadcrumbs and put them in a bowl. Chop the onion and pepper and add them to the bowl. Crack two eggs into the mix. Crush or finely mince the four cloves of garlic. Add the Italian seasoning mix and black pepper. Knead the mix and hamburger to an even consistency.

Spray your loaf pan with canola oil non-stick spray and put the meatloaf mix into it. Put the meatloaf into the oven for 50 minutes. If the top starts to blacken, remove from oven, carefully place an aluminum foil cover over it, and return it to the oven.

Remove from the oven. To reduce the fat content of the meatloaf even further, carefully tip it and drain the excess fat into an empty can.

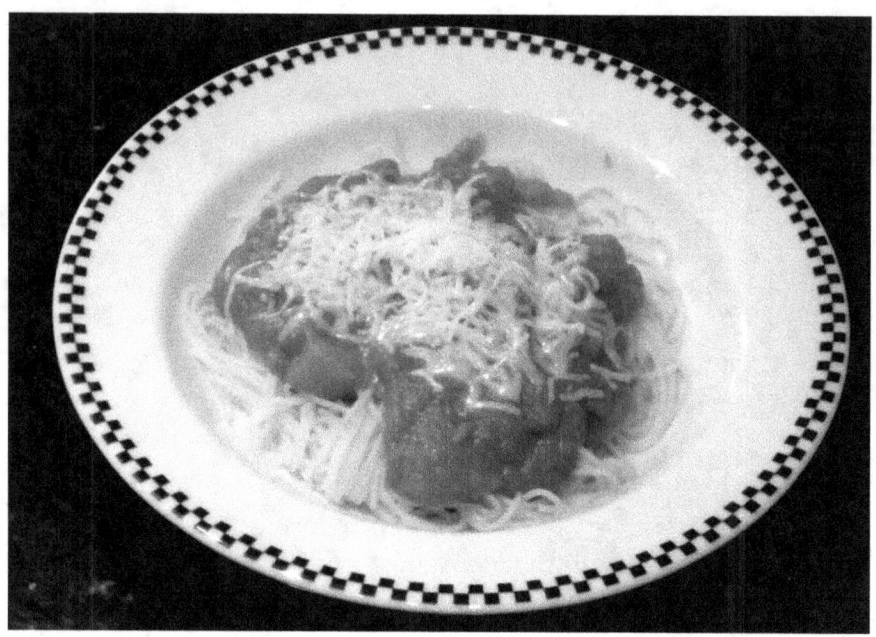

MARINARA SAUCE

Marinara sauce is incredibly easy to make and it's delicious and nutritious – especially compared with store bought sauces. This recipe has a lot of chunky green bell pepper, sweet red pepper, and onion, and a minute amount of olive oil. Two people should get at least ten servings out of this simple recipe.

Ingredients:

2   large cans crushed tomatoes

1   large can Hunts Tomato Paste

1   small can Contandina Tomato Paste

½   green bell pepper

½   sweet red pepper

1   Vidalia or yellow onion

1   head garlic

¼   teaspoon dried Italian seasonings

2   tablespoons olive oil

Instructions:

Pour the cans of crushed tomatoes and tomato paste into a large pan. Add 1/4 teaspoon of dried Italian seasonings and turn stove on medium.

Cut the green bell pepper, red sweet pepper, and onion into medium sized cubes. Put 1 tablespoon of olive oil and pepper and onion mix in skillet. Saute over medium heat until the onion begins to appear translucent. Add pepper mix to tomato sauce.

Peel garlic head. Mince or crush the garlic. Put 1 tablespoon of olive oil in skillet. Saute — do not brown — over medium heat. Add garlic to sauce.

Let the sauce simmer for a half hour, giving it a stir every five to ten minutes.

There you have it. Nutritious and delicious marinara sauce. Serve over the whole grain pasta of your choice.

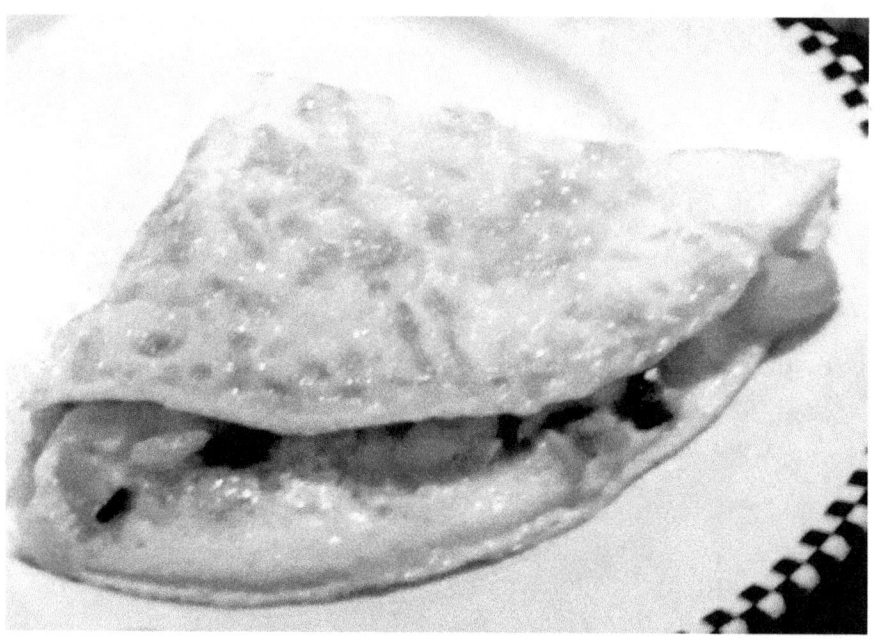

OMELET

Making an omelet is intimidating to many cooks, but it doesn't have to be if you follow this easy recipe for two.

Ingredients:

4   eggs (add another egg if you're using just the whites)

1   green bell pepper

1   sweet red pepper

1   Vidalia or yellow onion

1   jalapeno — Optional, and only if you like spicy hot food

1/4 cup shredded cheese — Italian blend or Mexican blend

2   teaspoons butter

Instructions:

Cut a quarter section from green bell pepper and sweet red pepper. Clean out the seeds and extra white parts. Dice the pepper sections and a quarter of the onion. Dice whole (optional) jalapeno — being careful to clean out the seeds. You should have a cup of vegetables.

Saute the vegetable mix in a teaspoon of butter over 1/4 heat. The vegetables are done when the onions start to appear translucent.

Crack four eggs and put in a bowl with a tablespoon of water. Whisk to even consistency.

Preheat a large skillet at 1/4 heat. Add teaspoon of butter and spread evenly over bottom of pan. Pour in egg mixture. When the egg mixture starts to solidify on the bottom — look through the bubbles — sprinkle the vegetable mix on one side of the egg mix and the 1/4 cup of cheese on the other.

Cover the large skillet and let cook for two to three minutes. Lift the pan top, the cheese should be melted and the eggs cooked — not runny. Take a spatula and flip the cheese half over onto the vegetable half.

There, you've made an omelet!

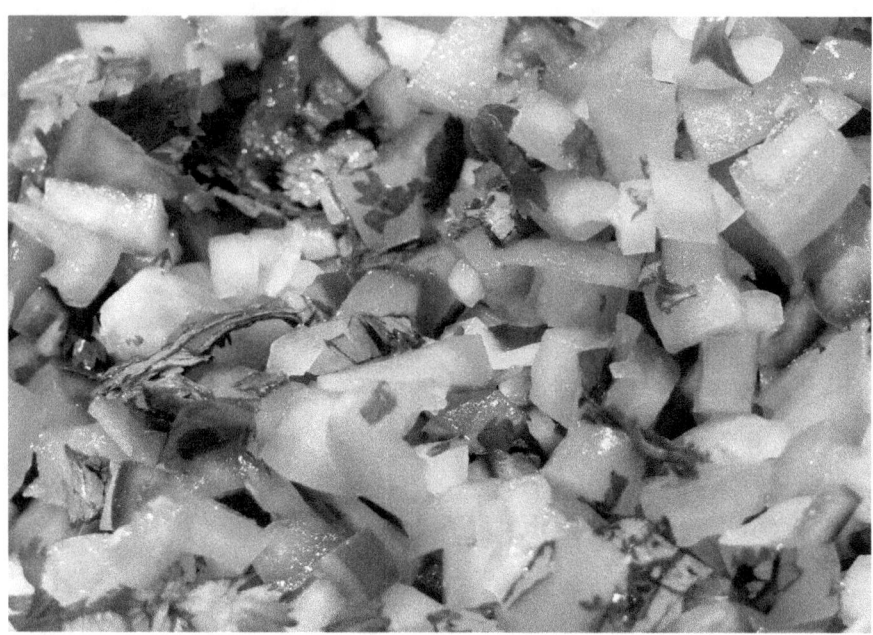

PICO DE GALLO (SALSA)

Pico de Gallo, a traditional Mexican salsa, has to be one of the healthiest snack foods. It's made of fresh vegetables, very little salt and no fat at all. Yet it tastes delicious on tortilla chips (baked and low salt, of course), tacos, enchiladas, Spanish rice, chicken, fish, and you name it.

Ingredients:

3   tomatoes

1   onion — yellow, Vidalia or red will do fine

1   lime

1   bunch cilantro — Make sure to check the tie if you buy it at the store. Nothing worse than getting home and discovering you bought parsley.

1/8 teaspoon or less salt

1/2 head garlic — optional

1   jalapeno

Instructions:

Cut tomatoes into quarter inch slices. Clean out seeds and core. Slice tomatoes slices into small pieces. Chop 1/2 of the onion into very small pieces. Remove the leaves from the cilantro stems and chop the leaves finer. Combine in a dish. Squeeze the lime onto the mix. Add 1/8 teaspoon of salt or less. This is all you need for the basic Pico de Gallo. If you like garlic and jalapeno, crush or mince the garlic into the mix and remove the seeds from the jalapeno and chop it into fine pieces. Stir both into the mix.

There you go, a delicious, nutritious, and easy snack food that you can eat guilt-free. Just be sure to serve it with low fat and low sodium tortilla chips or on other healthy dishes.

FINAL THOUGHTS

None of the diet recommendations in this book are ground-breaking, earth-shattering, or even exciting. They're not meant to be. Instead, they're proven and effective without forcing you to go without tasty meals.

We've all been too conditioned to believe natural foods prepared well aren't enough to provide our bodies with all the fuel they need to be healthy, when, in fact, for those of us without health conditions that need special attention, they are. Learn to play with your food – use your imagination and spices to make if fun, healthy, and tasty without harmful ingredients – and you'll be amazed out how much better you feel.

Lawrence S. Richardson, Jr.

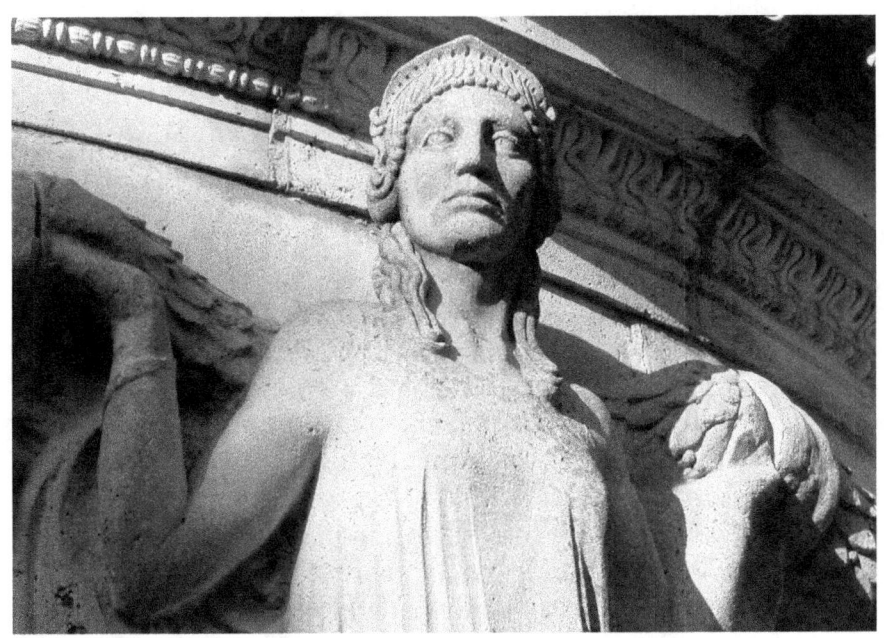

6 BRAIN BOOSTERS

Research has shown that exercise and a healthy diet both contribute to promoting a healthy brain as we age, which only makes sense. A brain that gets plenty of oxygen and essential nutrients pumped by a healthy heart through clean arteries and veins will age better than a brain that doesn't.

Increasingly, however, science is also finding that our brains benefit from challenging mental exercises and positive, nurturing social interaction. Brains that are stimulated in this manner tend to be:

➢ More alert.

➢ Better at processing information.

➢ Better at remembering people, events, and other information.

➢ Resistant to dementia and related diseases.

➢ At less risk of depression.

➢ More positive and possessing a heightened sense of well being.

Promoting brain health can be as simple as regular participation in mind-intensive puzzles and games -- including crosswords, bridge, chess, and stimulating video games – or reading books that force you to think. *(Go to Xeniors.com and enter the search word "reading" for a list of challenging classics and "brain" for the latest tips and tricks to promote brain health.)* Learning a foreign language, enrolling in adult education classes, or taking dancing lessons are also effective brain boosters.

If you want to really get your brain in gear and expand your horizons, consider taking up a completely new skill. For example, writing your life's story in a blog, capturing the world as you see it through photography or painting, or playing a musical instrument are excellent ways to stimulate your brain and get more out of life. This chapter features detailed tips to get you up and running in a handful of superb brain bolstering activities. There are certainly many more options out there for you to explore.

BEFORE YOU START

There are several important points to keep in mind when you're mastering a new mental skill, including:

➢ **Keep an open mind.** The fun and value of new skills is that they are not familiar to you. That means you have to be open to learning new information and techniques, instead of insisting that you already know how to perform them correctly before you begin.

➢ **Bring plenty of patience.** Patience is not only a virtue when learning new skills, it's essential. Learning something new isn't as simple as pouring information into your brain. If it were, we'd know everything without even trying – and where's the fun in that? Instead, you need to study the skill, practice it, and internalize it until you become proficient, all the while remembering that it could take a fair amount of time.

➢ **Be tenacious.** There are going to be times when learning something new becomes so challenging you will be tempted to quit. This is especially true when you have trouble understanding a specific piece of information or mastering a specific skill. It's these moments when you need to remember that working to break through a learning barrier is when your brain receives the greatest benefit. Often when you hit a wall, all you need to do is stop working on the skill for a little while and return with a fresh mind and take it on again. Hang in there, and you'll get it!

➢ **Exercise logic.** The best way to learn a new skill is to use logic. Our brains and bodies aren't able to take on something difficult and automatically do it. In most cases, it's up to us to break the information or technique down into small digestible units and practice them until we get it right. This is a logical and productive approach to learning that will keep you from becoming overwhelmed.

➢ **Be prepared to conduct research.** There are a wide variety of teaching approaches for most new skills. An approach that works for one person, might not work for another. If you hit a wall, don't keep running into it, do some research on the subject and see if there's another approach that might work better for you.

➢ **Put your spirit into the task at hand.** Once we master the classical mechanics of a new skill, we can make it our own by using our own inner self – our personality, thoughts and preferences – to express ourselves.

Using your spirit to make a skill your own is a truly fulfilling experience.

> **Feel pride about your accomplishments.** There's a certain satisfaction that comes from surmounting challenges on the way to mastering a new skill. The fact is most people drop out early when taking on a mental challenge. You should be proud of your accomplishments and be willing to share what you learn with anyone who has a similar interest. Remember, positive social interaction is also a brain booster. So anything you can do to help others will also help you to develop and maintain a healthy and happy mind.

BRAIN BOOSTING ACTIVITIES

The following brain boosting activities barely scratch the surface of what you can do to stimulate your mind and make it stronger. These suggestions are intended to help you begin to consider activities that truly interest you. That said, each of the activities on this list comes with detailed steps you can take today to get started. Enjoy!

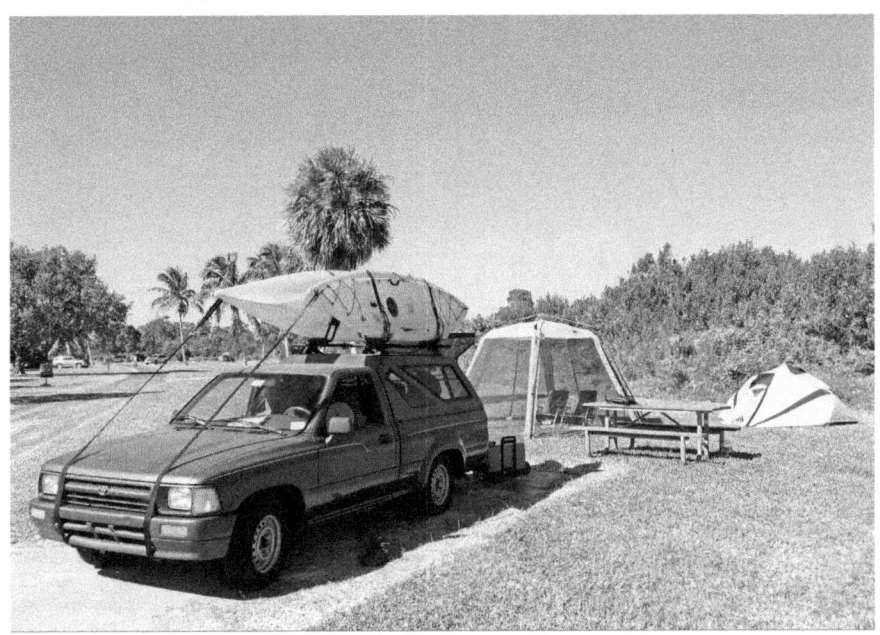

CAMPING

Camping might sound like an unusual choice for exercising your mind. But, when you think about it, there are a lot of details to work out before, during, and after an adventure. Living in the great outdoors involves a lot of exercise hauling gear, setting it up, and breaking it down, plus any hiking, biking, kayaking, or similar physical activity you decide to engage in. Add to that the challenge of using field guides to get to know an area's weather, geography, geology, flora, and fauna and you're really going to work your gray matter.

Before you go camping, you need to consider the following questions that will ensure you have a pleasant experience:

> **What type of camping do you prefer?** Are you going to stay in an RV, van, truck with a cap, pop-up camper, or tent? The answer to this question will determine the type of gear you need to bring along. RV camping is like traveling in a house so specialized outdoor gear isn't required. Tent camping, on the other hand, requires a

great deal of planning to ensure you're safe, comfortable, and protected from the elements. (There's a buyer's guide later in this section to explain the requirements in detail.)

➢ **What type of facilities do you prefer?** Are you going to stay at an RV park or campground with bathrooms, sinks, showers, and full amenities? Are you going to stay in a campground that has only a bathroom with a toilet and sink? Or are you going to rough it and hike out to a primitive campsite that lacks any facilities at all? The answers to these questions will impact the gear and amount of food and water you need to bring.

➢ **What type of environment are you camping in?** There's a huge difference between pitching a tent in Florida's Everglades National Park and staying at 8,600 feet in California's Yosemite National Park. The Everglades requires gear that can protect you from heat, humidity, rain, and swarms of mosquitoes, while Yosemite experiences such great extremes that heat, frigid cold, snow, and rain can all be issues during a single visit.

➢ **What activities are you going to participate in?** Hiking and kayaking obviously require different clothing, equipment, knowledge, and skills. Arriving prepared for your activities of choice will ensure you're safe and comfortable.

➢ **How many days will you stay?** This question is critical so that you bring enough food, water, and ice with you. Many campgrounds are limited in these necessities.

Now can you see how camping can be a brain-booster? Before you actually go camping, answer these questions by:

➤ Reading books and online articles about camping essentials.

➤ Visiting National Park Service and state park department websites to see what camping options are available in locations you intend to visit.

➤ Mapping out a trip and making reservations at campgrounds along the way.

10 QUICK CAMPING TIPS

1. **Practice setting up your tent and using your equipment before you go camping.** You don't want to find it's defective or missing a piece when you're in the middle of nowhere.

2. **Choose a campground that meets your needs.** Campgrounds range in amenities. Some have grand lodges, others have nothing but an outhouse. Find the campground that best fits your comfort level and call ahead to reserve a space. Be sure to ask what time the campground locks its gate, so you can make arrangements if you're running late.

3. **Bring cash, your checkbook, and a pen.** Some campgrounds don't accept credit. Also, budget extra cash for gas, food, and unexpected expenses.

4. **Ask the host for the campground rules.** They're also a great resource for tips on the weather, hiking trails, activities, and hazards.

5. **Know the climate of your camping location and bring appropriate clothing.** Some mountain campgrounds can be 80 degrees at noon and 40 degrees at night. A raincoat and rain pants can be especially helpful as rain and wind blocks. Also, having clothes

you can add and remove as needed. Good hiking boots will ensure you're comfortable in the great outdoors.

6. **Find a level area for your tent and clear it of debris that could pierce the floor.** This may take several minutes, but the investment is always worth it. Even a slight tilt to a tent floor can bring an uncomfortable night's sleep, and having a stick or sharp rock pierce your tent floor will open it up to critters and moisture.

7. **Be courteous to your fellow campers.** Don't use bright lights and electronic devices with the volume set at a level that will annoy other campers. Understand most people go camping to escape the distractions of modern life.

8. **Store your food in coolers and plastic boxes to keep out mice, ants, and other pests**. Be careful not to let your guard down. Critters are always on the lookout for a free meal. Also, put your food in bear boxes when required for your protection and the bears.

9. **Only light a campfire it it's allowed and you know how to manage it.** Have plenty of water and a shovel at the ready to extinguish the fire if it gets out of control or you're leaving. Don't leave until all the embers are extinguished.

10. **Bring your sense of humor.** Camping is supposed to be fun. The first few times out, you will have to spend extra time setting up and managing your campsite. Once you get the basics down, camping will be a breeze. Also, weather conditions can change rapidly, so be prepared and expect the unexpected.

ESSENTIAL GEAR

Mention camping and the first thing many people think of is lying in a leaky tent, wrapped up in a moldy, lumpy sleeping bag set on bone-grinding solid ground that leave you sleepless and praying for morning. Modern camping doesn't have to be like that at all.

Today's quality camping gear includes tents made of light weight, waterproof, synthetic materials with screened windows that can be left open to allow a cool breeze to blow through or shut tight to lock the heat in and the elements out. Sleeping bags have evolved to the point where they are comfortable in a wide range of temperatures, and they have evenly distributed fillers that prevent lumping and clumping. Add an inflatable sleeping pad into the mix, to provide a layer of cushioning between you and the ground, and you're in business.

Here are some general gear recommendations. *(Visit Xeniors.com and enter the search term "camping" for specific products.)*

1. **Tent.** Find a tent that:

    ➤ Is roomy enough for yourself and/or the number of people who will be camping with you.

    ➤ Light weight, especially if you're going to have to haul it.

    ➤ Has two or more zippered openings so you don't have to crawl over other people when Nature inevitably calls.

    ➤ Features a tough fly that can be thrown on top to keep out rain and cold. (Make sure the fly covers the entire tent. Some only reach half way down, which will be useless in blowing rain.)

> ➢ Includes a footprint, a polyester sheet that protects the tent bottom from direct contact with the ground.

2. **Sleeping Bag.** Buy a sleeping bag that:

> ➢ Is light weight and made of synthetic materials.

> ➢ Is rated for the temperature range you will be camping in.

> ➢ Has chambers that keep the insulating fill evenly distributed throughout the shell.

> ➢ Features a hood with draw cords, a draft tube that runs along the zipper to lock heat in and cold out, and a foot box that retains heat while letting your feet move freely.

3. **Sleeping Pad.** Buy a sleeping pad, a roll-up inflatable cushion that separates you and your sleeping bag from the ground, that:

> ➢ Is light weight and the right size for your body.

> ➢ Allows you to control the amount of inflation, which will determine the level of firmness.

> ➢ Is durable enough to stand up to abrasion from sand, small pebbles and twigs.

4. **Other Recommended Items:** Here's a list of optional items that will make your camping trip more enjoyable:

> ➢ Backpack for clothing and toiletries.

> ➢ Two-burner propane stove with extra gas canisters.

> ➢ Waterproof matches.

➤ Stowable pans, reusable plastic plates, bowls, and utensils.

➤ Large rollable cooler.

➤ Electric lantern and headlamp.

➤ Compressible pillow.

➤ Biodegradable dish soap and general cleaner.

➤ Microfiber towels.

➤ Insect repellant.

➤ First aid kit with instructions.

➤ Basic toolkit.

➤ Toilet paper and hand soap/sanitizer. (Often campgrounds run out of both.)

Beyond this list of essentials, you will need to prepare a shopping list that includes fruit, vegetables, snacks, and meals that can easily be prepared on a camping stove, grill, or over a fire. And, you must consider the clothing you will need to bring based on the climate and activities you plan to participate in. A good pair of hiking boots are always a must, as are a rain coat, rain pants, and quick-drying clothes. Bring backups too, in case you get soaked or you need to layer on clothes to deal with a sudden change in temperature.

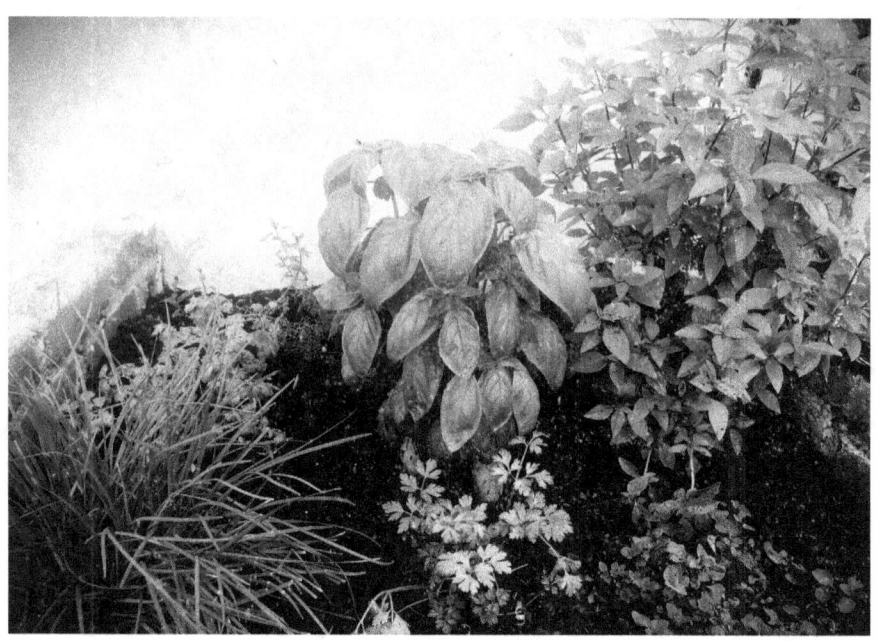

GARDENING

Gardening is great for your body, mind, and spirit. Your body gets plenty of exercise hauling around soil, watering, and weeding, and your mind gets plenty of exercise creating the right mix of sun, soil, water, and fertilizer to coax life out of the ground. When it all comes together, there's certainly something uplifting about tasting and sharing the fruits (and vegetables) of your labor.

To get plants to grow, you have to:

1. Choose an area of land or place to put containers – indoors or out – that receives just the right amount of sunlight for the types of plants you intend to grow.

2. Know when to plant each item based on its growing season.

3. Prepare the plot of land or containers, making sure to combine just the right mix of sand, soil, and fertilizer.

4. Know how often to water the plants.

5. Come up with a strategy to prevent pests from devouring your plants.

6. Recognize when the plants are ready for harvesting.

7. Find new and imaginative ways to prepare your fruits, vegetables, or herbs.

Many of us don't live in locations where it's practical to create a large garden. Fortunately, there are plants we can grow on a much smaller scale that still deliver an enormous return on investment. Herbs are an excellent example.

Even the tiniest garden can grow plenty of herbs for seasoning meat, poultry, fish, and vegetable dishes. If you've ever tasted fresh herbs, you'll know growing them is worth the effort.

If you're interested in herb gardening, there are many practical resources available at libraries, bookstores, and on the internet. It's a mental challenge to come up with the most productive plan based on your area's soil and climate.

7 Herb Gardening Tips

These herb gardening tips will help you to get started, but they are in no way the whole story. Solving specific problems as they arise is part of the mental challenge of gardening. To grow herbs you need to:

1. Decide whether you want to grow your herbs directly in the ground or in containers.

2. Prepare the soil mixture – potting soil and dirt – and make sure it drains properly.

3. Determine where to grow your herbs based on sun exposure. Some plants like lots of sun while others prefer shade.

4. Make sure they get adequate water and fertilizer.

5. Decide how you will deal with pests, which is relatively easy as most pests don't like herbs. Since herbs are delicate and you will consume the leaves, the less chemically-invasive approach you take the better. A light soap-based spray should get the job done.

6. Harvest the herbs in a way that doesn't completely deplete the plants.

7. Learn how to dry your herbs so you can enjoy them year-round.

Note: If seeds won't grow, try buying starter herb plants at a local nursery.

As you can see, there's a lot of work and problem solving involved in even the smallest garden, but the payoff is enormous. The first time you taste rosemary baked chicken, dill mashed potatoes, and summer squash sprinkled with parsley you grew yourself, you'll know what I mean.

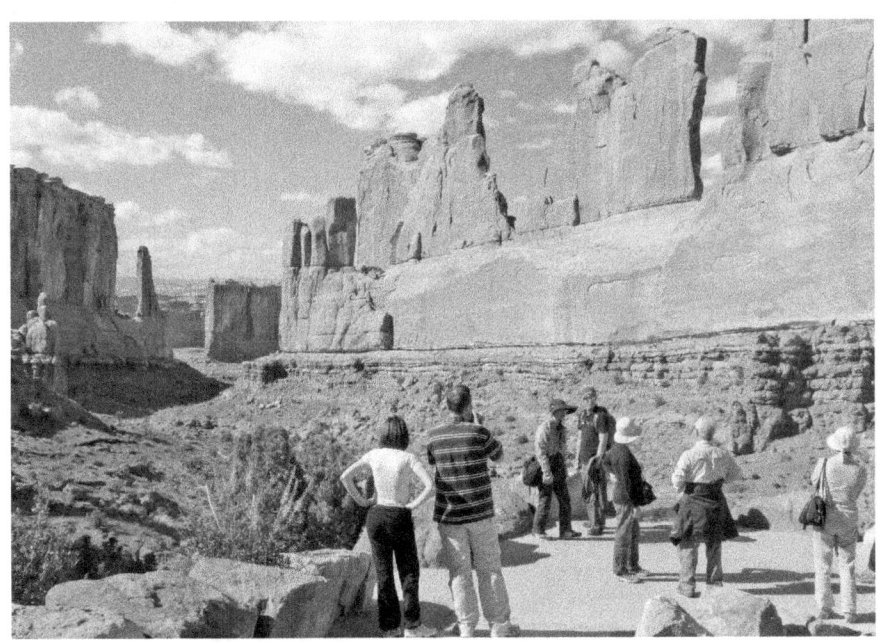

PHOTOGRAPHY

Photography is a terrific hobby for your body and mind. Going on a photo safari to find interesting subjects to shoot involves walking, hiking, and biking through cities, fields, forests, mountains, and beaches. When you find the perfect subject, you have to combine your knowledge of your camera and artistic eye to bring out its uniqueness and express how it makes you feel.

Fortunately, you don't have to have the latest, greatest camera to get the best shot. Digital cameras have been around for over a decade now, and yesterday's top shooter is today's supposedly obsolete discount model. An older, basic camera – or even a cell phone camera – in the right hands can yield excellent results if you follow a few simple tips. *(Visit Xeniors.com and enter "camera" or "photography" in the search window for camera buying recommendations and additional tips.)*

12 Photography Tips

The following basic photography tips will help you shoot great photos no matter what camera you're using:

1. **Go where the action is.** Great photos don't just happen. A huge factor is simply the subject you're shooting — be it a particularly colorful sunset, rolling surf, or field of wildflowers. Go out and hunt for a naturally attractive or interesting subject and you will create terrific photos.

2. **Use natural light.** In daylight hours outdoors, your camera flash will rarely yield as richly-colored photos as natural lighting. The only time you should use a flash in daylight is if you're shooting a person who is standing in an oddly shadowed location, like under a tree. Shooting without the flash in this situation can leave their faces covered with spidery shadows or with a background that's too bright and imposing. When you use your flash, make sure you're standing far enough from your subject that the flash of light won't completely wash them out. Indoors, too, regular room lighting – even if you have to switch on a few more lights – will usually yield better photos than firing your flash.

3. **Pay attention to composition.** In most situations, photographers follow the rule of thirds. An example: If you're shooting a person, try to frame them to the left or right third of the frame instead of directly in the middle. This rule is especially useful if you're shooting a person in beautiful scenery. If you're taking party pictures or portraits, the rule can certainly be broken. Try to frame landscape photos to get the most out of natural formations. Zooming in or out of your subject and panning from side-to-side and tilting up and down can make a huge difference in the results. For example:

Some fields of wildflowers look great as a broad carpet beneath a big sky while others are enhanced by zooming in on a handful of blooms. In ideal instances, your subject will look great composed in a variety of ways, so make sure to experiment. You can always delete the shots you don't like when you get home.

4. **Use a tripod.** Tripods are a must if you have a shaky hand, are shooting in low light situations where the shutter will be open for an extended period to collect enough light to produce an image, or using a powerful zoom lens. In all of these situations, your photo will be crisper with a tripod than if you shot it free hand. Tripods come in all sizes, weights, and quality. Find one that's sturdy but light enough to be carried around comfortably.

5. **Shoot lots of photos.** This is a pro-photographer's trick. Shoot a bunch of photos of your subject composed in many different ways, and you're bound to end up with a few masterpieces. You won't have to shoot as many as you become more familiar with your camera.

6. **Learn to set the exposure value (EV).** The exposure value lets you increase and decrease the brightness of a photo. (Shutter priority will also do this on more advanced cameras.) Find the EV feature in your camera menu and experiment with it. Understand that when you brighten a photo, your shutter will be open longer, so you have to have a steady hand or a tripod to avoid motion blur.

7. **Pre-focus the shot.** Most cameras have auto focus features. If you frame your subject and press lightly on the shutter release button, the auto focus will lock onto your subject. If you're satisfied with the clarity, press the button down fully and the camera will take the shot.

If not, reframe the photo and try again. You can also pre-focus the camera on your main subject and then with your finger still lightly pressing the shutter release button move the field of view right, left, up, or down to recompose the picture while your subject remains in focus.

8. **Know how to use subject metering.** Subject metering directs the camera to focus and set brightness levels based on the contents of an entire scene, a medium segment of the center of the scene, or a particular spot in the field of view. Spot metering is especially useful if you're shooting a specific subject within complicated surroundings, such as an animal in bushes or tall grass.

9. **Use the auto setting most of the time but know how to set the scene settings.** Most cameras are sold with an easy to find auto setting that is programmed to use electronic sensors to ensure your photo is in-focus, colorful, and bright. Also knowing how to use the scene settings will allow you to benefit from the experienced photographers and technicians who programmed your camera to help you to take great shots in specific situations, such as landscapes, low-light, outdoors, indoors, at sporting events, and in extreme close-up. As you become more proficient, you will advance to the point where you will want a more complex camera that gives you access to more advanced settings, such as shutter priority, aperture priority and full manual.

10. **Use optical zoom, not digital zoom.** Optical zoom uses your camera's lens to transmit light to your camera's sensor. Digital zoom uses electronics to focus light on a small portion of the sensor, which causes the quality to degrade. Make sure you know the point at which your camera's lens switches from optical to digital zoom – usually indicated by a colored bar on the viewing screen – and avoid it at all cost.

11. **Understand the importance of white balance.** Most cameras have an auto white balance setting. It enables the camera to shoot photos with natural looking colors in sunlight, clouds, incandescent light, and fluorescent light. Each of those light sources has a different color temperature, ranging from blue, to orange, to yellow. If you notice that you're getting unnatural looking photos – too blue, too orange, or too yellow in hue – you need to set the white balance for the type of ambient lighting you're under. If you have a camera that allows you to set the white balance manually, experiment until the color range matches the scene in front of you.

12. **Experiment, experiment, experiment.** In the age of film, photographers had to carefully consider every photo taken because film and processing were expensive. With digital photography, taking and viewing photos costs nothing. This frees us up to take as many shots as we want until we get the photo that expresses our artistic vision. Experiment with your camera's settings and see what works for you. That's what makes photography fun and interesting.

These basic photography tips are just a starting point for a very exciting hobby with limitless possibilities. Once you master the basics, you'll probably want to purchase a DSLR or DSLR-type camera with interchangeable lenses and more manual controls that will allow you to completely unlock your creative potential. If, despite this primer, you still don't know where to begin, you should consider taking an adult education class in photography or buying a bunch of books and diving in.

A final point about modern photography is that a lot of artistic effects that used to cost a fortune and take a lot of time to create, such as making a photo look like a sketch, a watercolor painting, or even stained glass, can now be performed with very basic photo-editing software. If your camera came with great software, give it a try. If not, take a look at Adobe Photoshop Elements. This affordable program will allow you to unleash even more of your creativity.

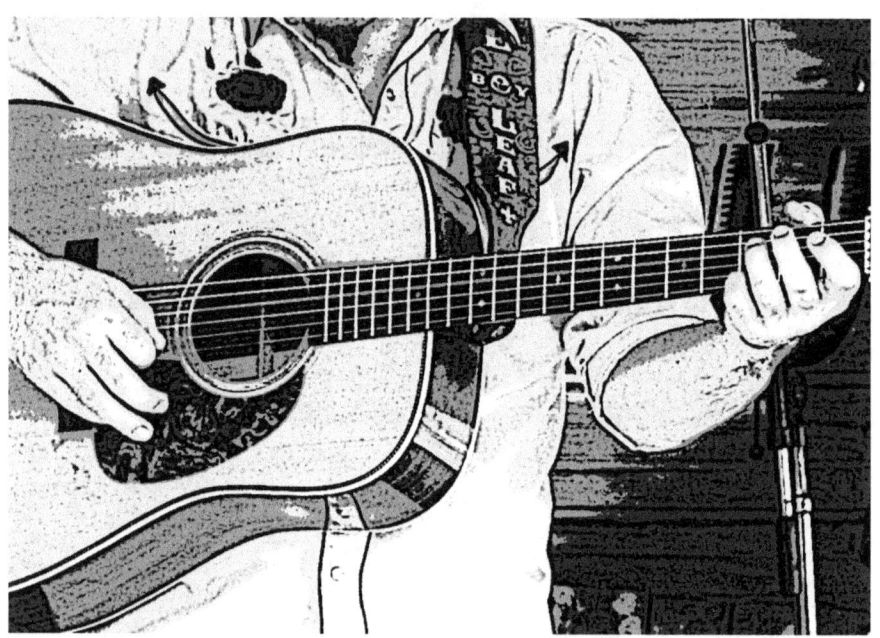

PLAY GUITAR

Whether it's listening to Joan Jett or Joan Baez, Eddie Van Halen or Elvis, at one point or another we all dream of becoming our favorite guitar hero. Guitar stars make playing guitar look exciting, enjoyable, and easy, and their every note sings to our souls.

In reality, for all but the rare prodigy, playing guitar is a long, arduous process, but one with enormous short and long-term rewards. Learning to play well requires the type of intense mental focus – to get your body to do what your brain's thinking – that builds strong minds and fine motor coordination.

To learn guitar, you have to spend hours practicing chords – the sound produced when one or more strings are depressed on the guitar neck and strummed – and scales – sounds produced when a series of notes that sound well together are played up and down the guitar neck – until your fingers literally bleed, especially in the first couple of weeks.

When you play your first song – and it actually sounds like it should – all the hard work will seem more than worth it, and you'll be eager to master more and more skills. The following tips will help you to get started. *(Visit Xeniors.com and enter the search word "guitars" for buying advice.)*

GUITAR PLAYING TIPS

Learning guitar can be a challenge but getting started doesn't have to be if you follow these basic tips. To learn how to play guitar:

1. **Select the type of guitar that fits your taste in music.** The main factor to consider when selecting a guitar is what type of music you like. People who like soft rock, country, and folk, as played by James Taylor, Johnny Cash, or Peter, Paul and Mary, tend to be drawn to all wood acoustic guitars. People who like rock and blues, as played, Peter Frampton, Thrash, or B.B. King, typically purchase electric guitars and amplifiers. You can, of course, cross between acoustic and electric, but when you're getting started you should keep it simple and choose the type of instrument that best suits your taste in music since you will be spending many, many hours with it.

2. **Try your guitar on for size.** When selecting an instrument, it's a good idea to go to an actual music store and try out the different makes and models that fall within your budget. Guitars fit your body differently depending on their design, and you want to buy one you can hold comfortably. Also, even within a specific make and model, some guitars sound better than others. So go in the store and strum away until you find a guitar that sounds appealing to your ear. Throughout this process, don't be pressured by salespeople. If it doesn't

feel or sound right in any way, don't buy it. You'll know when you find the right one.

3. **Don't go too cheap.** Cheap guitars, typically those priced under $250, can have a host of problems, the most obvious of which is the wood and workmanship are inferior – which causes them to deliver sub-par sound. Even worse than that, the tuners, the hardware that holds the strings taut, can be unreliable. If the tuners don't hold the strings firmly in place, you won't be able to tune your instrument. If the instrument is out of tune, it will sound bad even when you're playing good. Unfortunately, equipment failure is a top reason beginners become discouraged and quit.

4. **Purchase the other gear you need to get started.** Once you select your guitar, you will need to purchase a few other pieces of gear to play. Guitar picks can be slippery. If holding on to one is tough for you, consider purchasing a box of Snarling Dog Brain Guitar Picks. Both sides of the 1.00 picks are rough, which makes them easier to hold. Always have extra guitar strings on hand, too. Beginners usually have an easier time with lighter gauge strings that have more give. Strings have to be tuned to sound right. A chromatic headstock tuner that clips on to your guitar is the easiest way to pluck a string and see if it's in tune. If you're playing electric, you'll need to purchase an electric amplifier to hear what you're playing and headphones if you don't want to disturb others. There are many amps to choose from. Try to find one that fits the type of music you intend to play. A comfortable, armless chair, foot stand, and music stand are also helpful.

5. **Consider hiring a music instructor.** Once you make your guitar selection, it's time to decide your course of action. Literally. What type of course is right for you? Some people learn best from live instructors. When

you're in the music store picking out your guitar, check the bulletin board or ask around to find the best guitar teachers. Then audition them until you find one who is experienced, knowledgeable, inspiring, and within your budget.

6. **Consider learning from an instructional DVD set.** If an instructor is too costly, there are quite a few DVD-based courses that might be right for you. I tried a dozen bargain-basement DVD instructional videos and online tutorials before I found the perfect program for me: Gibson's Learn & Master Guitar. It's a comprehensive book, DVD, and jam-along CD collection by master-guitarist Steve Krenz that excels in many ways. Krenz, a friendly, accomplished instructor, starts at the very beginning. He shows you how to hold the guitar properly – you won't understand how important this is until one is swaying in your lap. Then he goes on to teach you the notes on each of the six strings and first three frets of the guitar and how to play chords in the same location. While you're learning the basics, he teaches you how to actually play simple songs. The first ten chapters of Learn & Master Guitar are so masterfully composed that by the time I finished I could play many pop, rock, country and folk songs — campfire style — without a hitch. The second half of Learn & Master Guitar involves music theory and specific genres that you can focus on as you advance as a musician. The bottom line is if you devote the time and effort to Learn & Master Guitar, you will live your dream of being able to play the challenging instrument.

7. **Be good to your body when you play.** Okay, you have a guitar and you have an instructional course, now the only thing missing is you. It's up to you to actually sit down and apply mental and physical effort to playing. As you work with the instrument, there are going to be times when you hit roadblocks. Many new players have

trouble with physical strain and difficulty relaxing enough to change notes and chords while keeping a steady strumming rhythm. Learn & Master Guitar addresses this to a point, but you may find you need more detailed instruction. Fortunately, accomplished guitarist Jamie Andreas has written books and produced DVDs that focus in on the minute details of playing guitar. Her materials tell you how to relax while you play, and they break every movement down – slow motion style – so you'll know where each finger should be when executing a note or chord change. Her basic theory is that if you practice each movement correctly in the beginning, you will become a great player. If you don't, you will be grabbing and grasping to sound each note and chord, and your poor foundation will disable you when you attempt to play more advanced material at a quicker pace. And she's right. Here are two books Jamie Andreas wrote that will help you to play in a healthy, relaxed, and productive manner: "The Principles of Correct Practice for Guitar" and "The Guitar Principles Path: Level One, Chords & Rhythm." You can buy either or both of them on Amazon.com. *(Please use the Amazon.com link on Xeniors.com.)*

8. **Purchase sheet music books with music you enjoy.** When learning how to play guitar, there are few experiences more satisfy than actually being able to play entire songs you enjoy. There are thousands of songs and song books to choose from. You should purchase books that include music with chords you already know and can play today – many songs consist of as few as three chords – and some chords you don't know so you have incentive to expand your chord library.

9. **Practice and play songs daily.** Set aside a half hour to hour a day for practice. Divide that time evenly between learning new skills, refining skills you've

already picked up, and playing songs you enjoy. The combination of the three will keep you headed in the right direction.

10. **Play with others.** The best way to improve overall is to play with others more advanced than you are. They will help you keep the proper rhythm and show you how to improve.

11. **Keep your guitar handy.** Guitars are made for playing. Put yours in a prominent place so you'll be tempted to pick it up and play every time you see it.

12. **Keep your fingernails trimmed extra short on your fretting fingers.** This piece of advice will seem strange to you until you actually play a guitar. Fretting requires pressing the strings down on the guitar neck with your fingertips. If your nails are long, they will get in the way.

13. **Remember to have fun.** Learning how to play guitar is, in many ways, difficult and at times it can be frustrating. That's when you need to take a break, cool off, remember it's supposed to be fun, and get back in there. Often a short break is all your brain and body will need to get it together.

As you can see, playing guitar is an excellent and rewarding challenge for your mind and body. If the guitar sounds too difficult, however, consider playing ukulele. It's much easier since it has four strings, not six like the guitar, and they're made of soft nylon, not metal. Not only that, most ukulele chords involve only one or two fingers. Read the next section for more information.

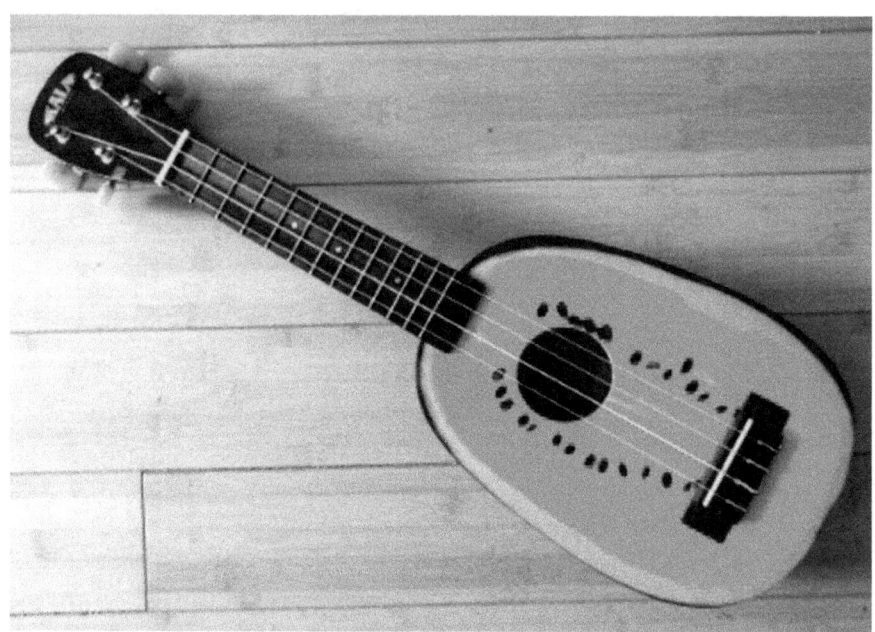

PLAY UKULELE

Musical instruments benefit your mind, body, and spirit. There are few instruments more perfect for beginners than the humble but lovable ukulele.

The ukulele is a small, light weight instrument with four nylon strings. Playing chords on a uke is as simple as pressing down on one string on a single fret (the space between two lines on the instruments neck) or as complicated as pressing all four strings on multiple frets while strumming with the fingernails on your other hand.

Learn how to strum with consistent rhythm while alternating between as few as two chords, and you'll be able to play many children's songs and a few popular hits. Learn a few more chords, and you'll be able to play many songs from the rock, country, folk, and other genres. *(Visit Xeniors.com and enter the search word "ukulele" for buying advice.)*

UKULELE PLAYING TIPS

The basic mechanics of playing ukulele sounds easy, but it still takes practice and dedication to do it right. The following tips will help you on your way. To learn how to play ukulele:

1. **Buy an instrument that suits your taste.** Ukuleles come in dozens of sizes, shapes, colors, and types. The most popular types are soprano and concert ukuleles. The soprano has the familiar jingly sound unique to the uke. The concert delivers a richer version of that sound. Plan on spending $50 or more for a ukulele. This is the price point where you'll start to see instruments that will actually stay in tune and sound good. The Lanikai LU-21CE/BK Concert Acoustic Ukulele is a sweet, modestly priced instrument that delivers rich sound on its own or plugged into an amplifier. Playing it as an electric instrument enables it to be heard when performing with other louder instruments.

2. **Buy other necessary gear.** Always have extra strings on hand to replace broken and worn strings that no longer stay in tune. You'll also need a chromatic headstock tuner for quickly tuning the instrument. And, if you go electric, you'll need a basic acoustic amplifier.

3. **Purchase an instructional DVD series.** Hiring an instructor for ukulele may be overkill. It's just not that complicated to play, and there are plenty of great books, CDs, and DVD sets available to give you all the instruction you need. "The Complete Ukulele Course for Kids!" is an excellent resource. It might sound like it's for wee ones, because it is, but it's also a fantastic instructional course to get adults started. Amiable host Ralph Shaw covers everything from buying a ukulele, to tuning it, to holding it properly. Then he shows you how to read ukulele music and create chords while

strumming. If you do what he says, you will be able to play the ukulele in no time.

4. **Buy a book of sheet music.** While you're learning how to play from instructional materials, you should keep a copy of "The Daily Ukulele" by your side. Liz and "Jumpin' Jim" Beloff have assembled 365 songs — traditional, folk, country, and rock — for all playing levels. The songs have chord charts — that show where to put your fingertips on the frets — sheet music, and lyrics.

5. **Concentrate when you're practicing, but also make sure to relax and have fun.** Playing ukulele is all about having a good time, and it's a journey. No points are deducted for mistakes or taking longer than you expected to master a skill. Relaxing and applying only as much force as is needed to strum or fret a chord will reduce the risk that you will strain your fingers, hands and shoulders.

6. **Trim your fingernails.** If you're right-handed, you need to grow nails on your right hand fingers to use when strumming. Cut your left hand fingernails all the way down so the fleshy part of your fingertips can press the strings into the frets to form chords.

7. **Go slow, real slow, when learning new chords, strumming patterns, or music.** The slower you go the better. As shaping the chords, strumming, and singing become easier, you can gradually speed it up. Starting fast and trying to make corrections will give you a foundation based on poor technique and actually lead to problems down the road as the music becomes faster and more complex.

8. **Pay attention to the relationship between chords.** Understanding the similarities between chords as you

move from one to the next will allow you to save time and go with the flow in a more natural way. For example, moving from an A chord to an F chord requires moving one finger, not both.

9. **If you are rhythm challenged and can't instinctively follow a beat – like many people – use a metronome to count out the beats for you.** Start the metronome out slow and gradually speed it up. As you get faster, play along with recordings of your favorite songs to master staying in synch.

10. **Learning to read music is difficult at first, but it's worth the investment in time and effort.** Take the time to understand at least the basics of reading music, and you will be able to play from many different types of sheet music.

11. **Play music you love.** The more passionate you are about the music you play, the quicker you'll learn and the better you'll sound.

12. **Play with others as often as possible.** You will progress faster as a musician if you practice and play with others. They will help keep you on the beat. Even better: Their friendship and support will provide another enriching aspect of your journey as a musician.

There are many instruments to play, but few are as accessible as the ukulele. It will give you a comprehensive understanding of musicianship that can easily be transferred to more complex instruments, including guitar, mandolin, and banjo.

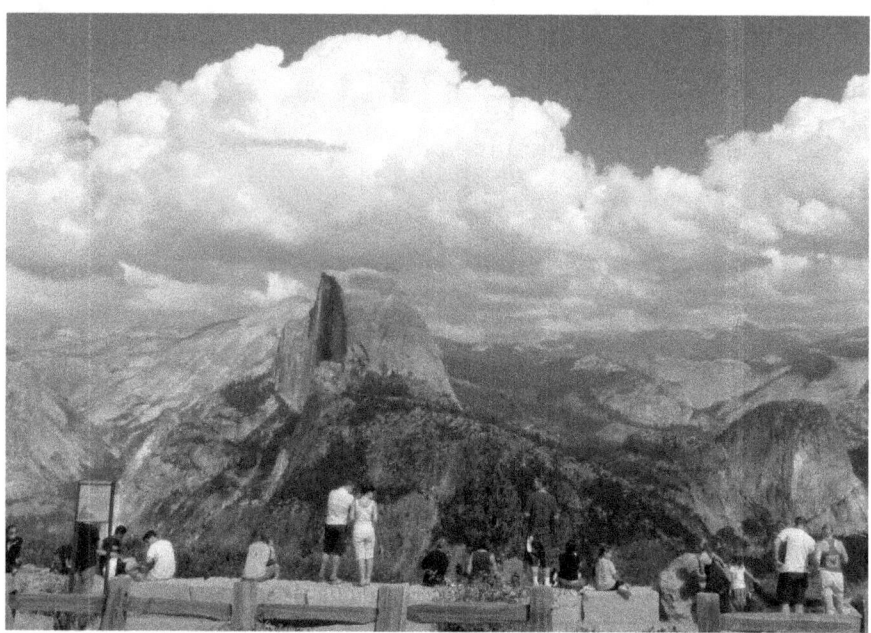

VIDEOGRAPHY

With the price of cameras capable of shooting high quality video plummeting, more and more people are becoming involved in videography. Shooting and editing video is a great way to exercise your brain, express your creativity, and log aerobic miles hiking in search of subjects. In addition, video cameras and still cameras that also shoot video are becoming so inexpensive and easy to operate you no longer need to go to school to create masterpieces. *(Go to Xeniors.com and enter the search word "video" for videography tips.)*

VIDEO SHOOTING TIPS

Here are some video shooting tips to help you get started:

1. **Purchase a camera that shoots HD (high definition) video, which looks great on computer screens and TVs**. There are many affordable cameras that shoot photos and videos or just videos. Cameras small enough

to fit in the palm of your hand are now capable of recording amazing video clips.

2. **If you're going to interview people, buy a video camera with a dedicated microphone jack.** A microphone that's held near the mouth of the subject will always yield better results than a camera-mounted microphone.

3. **Choose any event or subject that interests you.** Documenting your life might not seem interesting to you, but if you handle it with honesty and artistic flair, it will hold your viewers' interest and have lasting value. Going outside your own life's experience and covering events or adventures in your town or around the world can also be very fulfilling for you and your viewers.

4. **When you're shooting video, try to find areas with adequate lighting to avoid creating dark footage.** Either shoot outdoors or in a well-lit area indoors. You can turn up indoor lighting to suit your needs. Some dedicated video cameras also come with hot shoes so you can attach a light. Still, natural outdoor or room lighting always looks better than glaring camera light.

5. **If you have trouble holding a camera still, use a tripod or lean against a wall or other solid object for support.** Shaky video is hard to watch, so do everything you can to stabilize the camera while shooting.

6. **Don't zoom in and out, pan (move from right to left) or tilt (look up and down) too often unless your subject is hyper-active.** Rapid camera motions can lead to distorted video and viewer fatigue.

7. **Remember sound is as important as the picture.** In fact, video websites have found that people will forgive a poor video image more readily than poor sound. Get close to your subject to ensure good sound quality, or use a separate microphone.

8. **When you're considering how best to frame your subject, take a look at the background, too.** Make sure the background's not so distracting that people will focus on it instead of your subject.

9. **Shoot short – under a minute – video clips.** Short video clips are much easier to sort and edit than long clips.

10. **When you're editing and assembling your video clips into a completed video, pick the absolute best clips to represent the way you witnessed the event and throw away the rest.** As video proliferates, viewers are becoming more demanding. They want to be entertained, and they have little patience for boring or poorly edited clips.

In addition to purchasing a good camera, it's important to consider what type of computer and video editing software you will use. Desktop computers provide the most power for video editing, which often involves large files that demand a lot of memory and processing ability. However, if you need to edit away from home, there are powerful laptops that are up to the job. Read video editing websites for the latest recommendations.

VIDEO EDITING TIPS

The true art of video editing is cutting and reassembling clips in a way that keeps your audience interested. Your family might want to see long videos of private gatherings or sporting events but strangers will most likely want to see only the highlights. Even the most basic editing programs will allow you to:

- ➢ Cut the boring parts out of your videos.

- ➢ Rearrange the interesting video clips in any order you like.

- ➢ Add titles and transitions – such as fading in and out of clips.

- ➢ Add narration from a track you record on a handheld recorder or directly into your computer using an external microphone.

- ➢ Add a soundtrack with music – preferably performed on your ukulele, guitar, or other instrument.

- ➢ Automatically upload the video to video sharing sites, such as YouTube and Vimeo.

When creating videos for yourself, your friends, your family, and the world, using these general video shooting tips will help you to express your artistic mind while producing videos people will actually want to watch.

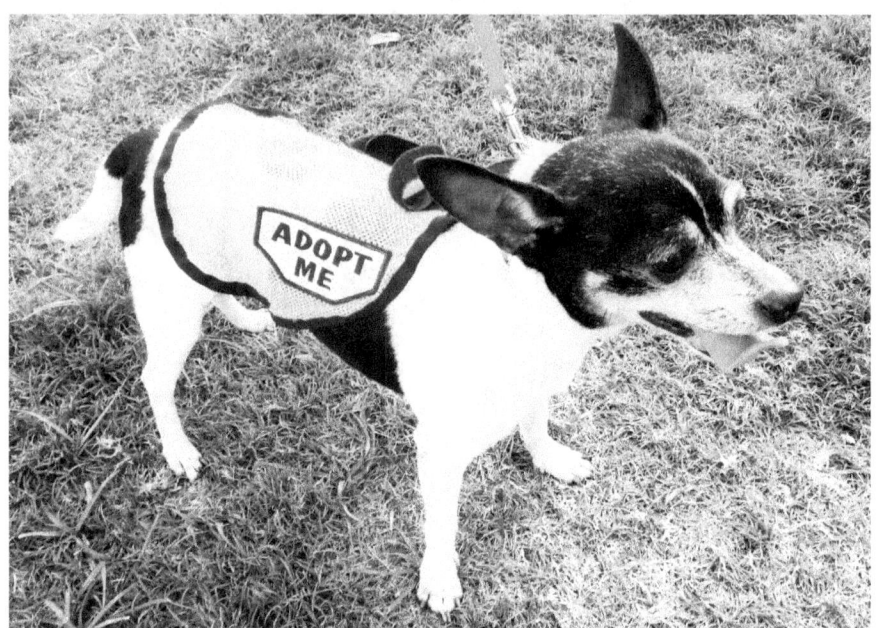

VOLUNTEER

Volunteering challenges your mind and body by presenting new skills to learn, encouraging you to leave your home and be physically active, and promoting interaction with people who want to make a positive difference in the world. Dedicating yourself to serving others is such a powerful elixir the positive benefits are scientifically measurable.

In 2013, researchers at Carnegie Mellon University reported that older adults who volunteered 200 hours of work a year were 40 percent less likely to develop high blood pressure. They reached this conclusion after surveying over 1,000 adults between 51 and 91 years in age with normal blood pressure in 2006 and then again in 2010. During the second session, they found that the active volunteers were less likely to report high blood pressure as a health condition.

The researchers reported that the type of volunteer work didn't matter as much as the volume. They theorized that positive social interaction was the force that made a huge difference in a volunteer's health.

TIPS FOR VOLUNTEERING

An enormous number of local, state, and national organizations are constantly seeking volunteers. If you're interested in improving your health while brightening the lives of others, here's how to get started:

➢ **Research organizations that enlist the help of volunteers**. Local hospitals, places of worship, public food pantries, the Veterans Administrations, senior centers, Meals on Wheels, the American Red Cross, and animal shelters are great places to start. You can find contact information in the phone book or online.

➢ **Contact the organizations of interest.** Arrange an appointment to meet with the volunteer coordinator to discuss opportunities of interest to you.

➢ **Meet with the volunteer coordinator.** Be prepared to discuss any skills you may have that will help the organization to serve the community. Also, be open to unfamiliar opportunities that will give you a chance to learn new skills.

When you begin working your actual assignment, be friendly, positive, professional, and cooperative, and soon you'll be a valued member of the volunteer team.

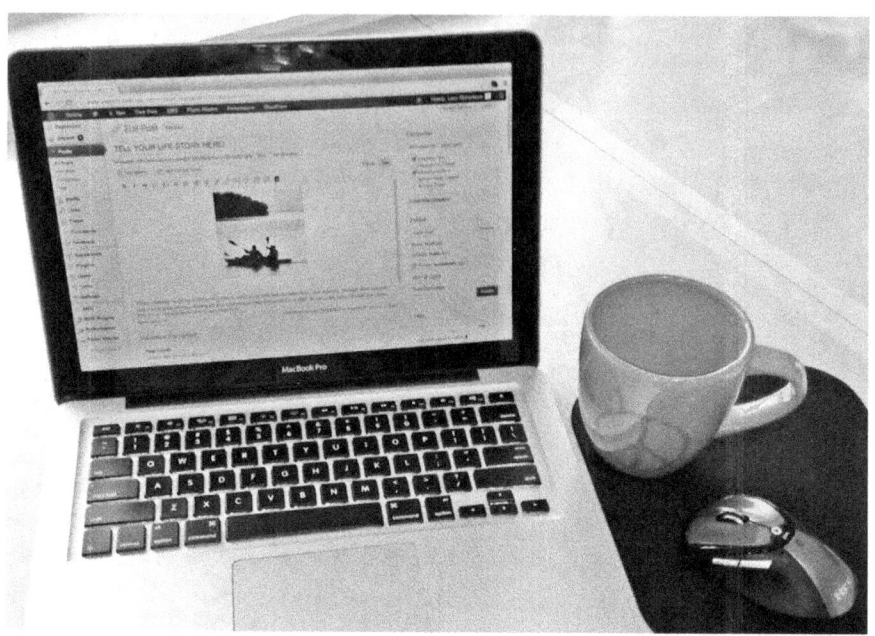

WRITE A BLOG

Writing is an amazingly effective way to exercise your entire brain. When you write, you actively engage the sections of your brain responsible for language, creativity, memory, logic, and analytical skills to organize your thoughts into a coherent narrative.

A fantastic way to practice writing is to tell your friends, relatives, and the world about your life by creating an online blog – or journal – that recounts your past and shares your everyday experiences. Don't be intimidated by the strange word "blog" – we'll get to the simple steps of creating one in a moment.

You might not see the value in setting up a blog and sharing your thoughts and experiences right now, but it's there. Most of us don't know much more than a few humorous stories about our own parents, let alone our grandparents and other forebears. But when we find a scrap of paper, even something as basic as their birth certificates, it means a lot to us.

If simple facts like birth date and location have significance, imagine how much your friends and relatives (today's and generations down the line) will value reading your story in your own words. Letters, diaries, and journals have enormous value and increase our understanding of the world in which we live, but few exist compared to the number of people who have inhabited the earth. Writing a blog is an opportunity for you to explain how you see the world and add your voice to human history.

HOW TO CREATE A WORDPRESS BLOG

Creating an online blog is easy and it's free. There are a number of blog-hosting sites, but Wordpress.com is among the easiest and most versatile. The following steps for signing up with Wordpress.com were current when this book was written. The Wordpress.com site has always been easy to navigate, so any changes since then shouldn't create a problem.

1. **Sign up for a free account.**

   ➤ **Go to WordPress.com**: Enter "WordPress.com" in your browser window, hit enter, and the homepage will appear.

   ➤ **Click "Get Started."** You will be taken to a screen with fields to be filled in. Don't be intimidated. It's actually quite easy.

   ➤ **Blog Address**: Fill in the blog address you would like to use. For example, it can be as simple as your name – JohnSmith or JohnSmithsStory – or as fanciful as MyWonderfulLifeInKentucky. It's totally up to you.

   ➤ **User Name**: WordPress automatically fills in your user name based on your blog address, but here too, you can choose to use a totally different name by deleting the name that's there and filling in the user name you would like to use. You need your user name to sign in to WordPress.com. So write it down.

> **Password**: Enter a password with numbers, letters, and symbols. Make sure you write your user name and password down because you will need them every time you log in to write a post. Confirm your password. Important Note: Passwords are case-sensitive. That means if you use a capital letter or a small letter in your password, you have to use a capital letter or a small letter when you sign in to your WordPress.com blog account.

> **Email Address**: Enter the email address you currently use. Double and triple check that you entered it right. WordPress.com will send an email to this address asking you to confirm that you want to set up a blog.

> **Consider Upgrading to a Paid Account**: If you intend to write a blog with text and the occasional photo, stick with the free blog. If you intend to publish a blog with lots of photos, videos, and other media, it's a good idea to pay for the upgrade. Since you're just getting started, the free blog should be more than adequate. If you want to stay with the free blog, click "Create Blog."

2. **Write and design your permanent information**.

> **Update Your Profile**: While you wait for WordPress.com to send you an account activation email, you can write your blog profile. Enter your first name and last name (or a pen name), then write an autobiography with as little or as much detail as you like. **Important Note**: Only include information you're comfortable with the whole world seeing. Never include your home address, phone number, social security number, or any other identifying information that can create problems if it falls into the wrong hands.

➢ **Activate Your Blog**: Check to see if the WordPress.com account activation email has arrived. If it has, open it. When you **click** "Activate Blog" in the email, you will be taken to your new blog page. Congratulations, you're a blogger!

➢ **Choose a Theme**: A theme is the basic graphic design – the colors, the print size and type, and the style – of your blog. The cool thing about WordPress.com is whether you've been blogging for minutes or years, you can switch to an entirely new theme with a single click. Review the themes presented on this page. Some are free and some cost money for lifetime usage. Until you're comfortable with the Wordpress.com interface, you should go to the bottom of this page and click "No thanks, I'll just stick with the default theme for now."

➢ **The Dashboard Page**: The Dashboard page is where you manage your blog's appearance, performance, and content. It can be as simple or as complicated as you want to make it. The simple approach is as easy as clicking on the left side of the dashboard where it says "Posts." This is where you will write the first entry in your blog.

➢ **Post Your Story and Thoughts**: To make your first post, click on "Posts" in the upper left side of the WordPress.com dashboard screen. You will be given a choice of clicking on "All Posts," which shows the posts you've already made. Or "Add New," which brings up the screen you use to post new stories or thoughts. Click "Add New." At the top of the post screen, there's a long box. Fill the title of your post in here. It can be something like "Welcome to my new blog!" In the rectangle below, you can fill in your story and thoughts. There are several tools you can use to format your font and paragraphs in the box above the posting field. The "ABC" field with the check will activate the spell checker. Remember: It's your blog so you can write anything you like – from old family stories to personal experiences to your thoughts on the world. Just be careful not to insult or lie about anyone still alive who is not a public figure. If you do, you could be sued for libel. Also, remember that while it's good to use proper spelling and grammar, they shouldn't keep you from expressing yourself. Sharing what you think is more important. Some of the most authentic and interesting histories are written in fractured grammar that only adds to their charm.

➢ **Publish Your Post**: Once you're through writing down your ideas, you can put your post out for all to see by clicking the "Publish" button on the right side of your screen. If you don't like what you wrote, you can edit it or click "move to trash" to delete it at any time.

➢ **View Your Blog and Posts**: To view your blog and posts, put your cursor over your blog name in the upper left hand corner of your dashboard screen. A drop down menu will say "Visit Site." Click "Visit Site" and another window will open with your actual blog as the public sees it. Impressive!

➢ **Edit Your Posts**: If you're not happy with your post, go back to your dashboard window, click on "Posts," then "All Posts." Your posts will appear in blue. If you put your cursor over the title of the post you want to change, "edit" and "delete" will appear below the title. Click "edit" and your post will appear in its entirety. Once you're done editing it, click "Update" on the right side of the screen and the improved version will appear on your blog. At any point, you can click "delete," and the post will be removed from public view.

➤ **Save a Draft**: If you're working on your blog and get interrupted, click "Save Draft" in the right side column on your screen. When you sign back in at WordPress.com using the user name and password you created earlier, you will be taken to your dashboard. Click "Posts" then "All Posts" and you'll see the title of the post you were working on. Put your cursor over the title and "edit" will appear. Click on "edit" and you can resume working on the post. When you're done, click "Publish" on the right side of the screen, and your post will be published on your blog.

➤ **Include Photos in Your Posts**: If you have photos stored on your computer that you want to include in your post, put your cursor where you want the photo to appear in your blog – top, bottom, or anywhere else – and click. Then move your cursor to just above the box where you were writing and you'll see "Upload/Insert" with a photo and musical notes. Click on this and a screen will open that asks you to browse your computer's files for the photo you want to use. Find the photo file name and click it, and it will be uploaded to the place in your post where you left your cursor. Note: When possible, resize your photo to a smaller size, this will take up less memory in WordPress.com computers and make your blog page download faster on visitor's computers.

3. **Keep learning more about effective blogging.**

➤ **Explore and Grow**: Once you have a basic understanding of WordPress.com, you can change the appearance of your blog on the dashboard by clicking "Appearance" in the left hand column and then "Themes." Take a look at the many free and paid themes WordPress offers. You can activate the theme or preview it to see what your blog will look like with the new theme. Other buttons in the left-hand column allow you to customize WordPress to the extreme and add many features — photo albums, videos, music, and Web page links — that will make your site more interesting.

➢ **Read About Effective Blogging:** Worpress.com offers outstanding tutorials on blogging on its website. The best book I've found that provides an easy to understand guide to blogging is unfortunately named "WordPress for Dummies." Despite its name, it offers many valuable blogging tips and tricks.

➢ **Read Others' Blogs:** You can search WordPress.com to find others' blogs. When you find blogs that interest you, subscribe to them and invite the auhtors to subscribe to your blog. This is how you can build a community of bloggers who will hopefully read your blog and post comments.

***One final important technical note: Inexperienced computer users should use WordPress.com. Experienced computer users with more than a casual understanding of how the internet works should consider registering their blog with WordPress.com's sister site WordPress.org. WordPress.org allows you to use your own domain name without the WordPress extension, place your blog on your own site hosting service, and greater customizing options. Visit both WordPress.com and WordPress.org and decide which platform you want to use before you register.

FINAL THOUGHTS

Our minds crave and need exercise every bit as much as our bodies do, and both gain substantially from new, challenging, and stimulating experiences. The secret to a fit mind is finding activities that you're truly passionate about that will inspire you for a lifetime. Activities you can share with others will deliver even more benefits, as socializing with others with a common interest has been shown to increase mental fitness.

Lawrence S. Richardson, Jr.

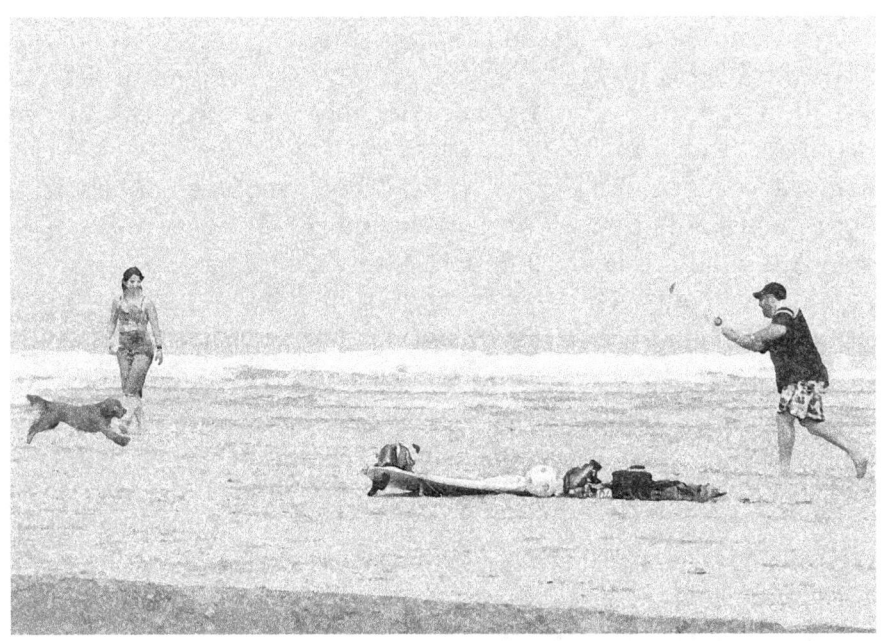

7 SPECIAL HEALTH CONDITIONS

According to the U.S. Centers for Disease Control and Prevention (CDC), chronic diseases – including heart disease, stroke, cancer, diabetes, arthritis, and obesity – are the most common and preventable of health problems. The majority of Americans report having a chronic disease. Two in three of us are obese or overweight.

The CDC blames most of these chronic conditions on four modifiable behaviors:

1. Lack of physical activity.

2. Poor nutrition.

3. Tobacco use.

4. Excessive alcohol consumption.

We've already discussed the important role physical activity and eating a healthy diet play in promoting our overall fitness. We didn't get into smoking and alcohol abuse because they're problems that obviously have to be solved before you can achieve maximum fitness, and they require specialized approaches outside the scope of this book.

This chapter is intended to show people with the most common chronic health conditions that they can still achieve fitness through an exercise program that accommodates their health challenges. Fortunately, organizations dedicated to combatting chronic diseases have created resources to help people with a wide range of conditions to improve their health by becoming more active.

GET STARTED!

GET YOUR PHYSICIAN'S PERMISSION!

As you've seen elsewhere in this book, before you begin a fitness program, **you absolutely must seek your physician's permission and guidance.** This step is especially important when you have a chronic condition that may actually be made worse by engaging in certain exercises.

For example, a person with heart disease may need special instructions to even begin walking to avoid putting too much stress on their cardiovascular system. People with high blood pressure may be advised to avoid certain exercises – such as weight lifting – that may cause their blood pressure to spike. And people with diabetes may be given special instructions to ensure their blood glucose level remains in a healthy range when they're exercising.

Your physician and physical therapist, if you're working with one, are your best sources of information and advice when you're contemplating a fitness program. They can:

➤ Evaluate your current condition.

➤ Tell you how to safely warm up before exercising.

> ➢ Advise you on specific aerobic and strength training exercises that will be productive and those you should avoid based on your health condition and any medications you are taking.

> ➢ Provide instructions on how to recognize problems that may develop before, during, and after exercise and how to deal with them.

> ➢ Refer you to specific facilities, gyms, and personal trainers who know how to accommodate your type of chronic disease.

DECIDE IF YOU NEED A PERSONAL TRAINER

People with chronic conditions can benefit greatly from adding a certified personal trainer to their team of healthcare professionals. A personal trainer who is qualified to instruct them in a way that accommodates their specific health challenges can help them to improve their overall health and reduce further complications. Specifically, a personal trainer can:

> ➢ Work with your physician and physical therapist to design a productive fitness program that won't exacerbate your condition.

> ➢ Conduct appropriate tests to determine your fitness level, which will act as a guide in designing your fitness program.

> ➢ Work with you to choose appropriate exercises you enjoy and then ask for your physician's or physical therapist's approval.

> ➢ Help you to warm up, exercise, and cool down in a way that takes your chronic condition into consideration.

➢ Monitor your health throughout an exercise session and provide guidance to ensure you are able to exercise with proper form and control.

➢ Assist you in the event of an unexpected medical emergency or less serious complication.

➢ Help you to overcome any anxiety you may feel about becoming more active.

➢ Motivate you to stay in the game by charting your progress and rewarding your achievements.

Certainly, in some cases, your physician or physical therapist will give you permission to exercise without a fitness trainer, but it's good to know this option is available.

GENERAL PRECAUTIONS AND RESOURCES

Providing detailed advice to help you exercise with a physical challenge is beyond the scope of this book. This section is meant to give you a general idea of the type of advice physicians, physical therapists, and personal trainers give to help people exercise who have a chronic condition and to encourage you to further explore your fitness options. It also has contact information for health organizations that can provide further information. *(Inclusion of an organization in this section is not an indication of an endorsement or relationship between the author and the organization.)*

1. **Arthritis**

Millions of Americans suffer from arthritis, a disease that affects joints, tissues around a joint, and other connective tissues. The most common version, osteoarthritis, occurs when cartilage, which provides cushioning between bones, breaks down and a bone is no longer able to glide over another. As a result, the individual experiences pain, swelling, and stiffness. In many cases, a lack of exercise can actually cause a person to experience greater degeneration, pain, and immobility.

To mitigate the effects of arthritis, experts recommend that people with the disease participate in light-to-moderate exercise. This can include aerobic activity, such as walking, swimming, dancing, or riding a stationary bike, two or three days a week, and strength training another two or three days a week. They should not work out to the point of fatigue and adjustments to intensity should be made based on how well they feel on a given day.

Pre-workout preparations are especially important for people with arthritis. The Arthritis Foundation recommends that they use heat to get their bodies ready for exercise. Specifically, they can benefit from taking a long warm shower or bath then wearing layered clothing that will keep their bodies warm but that can be peeled off as they become even warmer during exercise. Also, if any warm-up exercise or stretch causes pain, the activity needs to be eliminated or modified to avoid causing further harm or causing the person to quit their fitness program.

People with arthritis often experience pain after an exercise session. This can be alleviated by applying cold therapy, such as a bag of ice wrapped in a towel or a gel-filled cold pack for around ten minutes.

Useful Resource: Arthritis Foundation at www.arthritis.org

2. Cancer

According to the American Cancer Society, more than a million Americans are diagnosed with cancer each year. Cancer, a group of over 100 diseases, occurs when abnormal cells grow out of control.

With so many types of cancer, peoples' bodies are affected in many different ways. The Cancer Society recommends that people with cancer continue to exercise as much as their doctors recommend. Exercise helps them to maintain strength, flexibility, mobility, breathing, and appetite. It also helps control anxiety and relieve fatigue.

Useful Resource: American Cancer Society at www.cancer.org

3. Diabetes

Diabetes occurs when a person's body cannot regulate blood sugar levels. The body needs blood sugar to fuel cells, but too much can be harmful. People with diabetes have to modify their diet and/or take medications to control their blood glucose (sugar) level.

According to the American Diabetes Association, physical activity is also key to managing the condition. Exercise makes cells more sensitive to insulin, the chemical our bodies create to control blood sugar levels, so it can work better. Furthermore, with exercise, the cells themselves become more efficient at using and removing blood glucose.

People with diabetes must work with their physicians to identify appropriate exercises. But, in general, they can participate in the same aerobic and strength training activities as non-diabetics as long as they don't have serious complications that can occur with diabetes, such as heart disease, vision problems, or nerve problems. Even in cases where these complications are present, physicians should be able to help people with diabetes find exercises that can be performed safely.

People with diabetes do however have to take some special precautions, such as:

➢ Checking their blood glucose level frequently before and after exercise to understand how it is affecting their bodies and what they need to do to keep it in a safe range while working out.

➢ Having a fast-acting carbohydrate – for example a sugary sports drink, fruit juice, or soda – handy in case their blood glucose level plummets and they become hypoglycemic.

➤ Exercising with a personal trainer or buddy who can help them in an emergency.

Useful Resource: American Diabetes Association at www.diabetes.org

4. Heart Disease

There are several types of heart disease. The most common are atherosclerosis – plaque buildup in artery walls – heart failure, irregular heartbeat, heart attack, and stroke. The American Heart Association recommends that people with heart disease partner with their doctors, nurses, pharmacists, and other health care professionals to create an exercise plan that will help them to become healthier and reduce the risk of future problems.

The Heart Association recommends that, with their physician's approval, people follow the general health guidelines and get at least 150 minutes of brisk aerobic exercise a week and two or more strength training sessions a week. Special precautions usually include exercising with a physical therapist or personal trainer who is familiar with their medical condition and who can monitor their heart rate and blood pressure throughout a session to make sure they remain within a safe range. They should also be careful to breath properly while exercising, maintain a relatively relaxed grip on handles and other exercise equipment, and not remain still while exerting themselves, all of which will help keep their blood pressure in a safe range.

The Heart Association also recommends that people with heart disease watch for warning signs that indicate they are working too hard or experiencing a heart attack, such as squeezing, burning, or heaviness in the chest that spreads to the left shoulder, back of the throat, or jaw, lightheadedness, dizziness, or confusion, nausea, extreme fatigue after exercise, unusual shortness of breath, or fast or uneven heartbeat. If they experience these symptoms, they need to stop exercising and call their doctor or 9-1-1 right away.

Useful Resource: American Heart Association at www.heart.org

5. High Blood Pressure

Over 75 million American adults have been diagnosed with hypertension, or high blood pressure, according the American Heart Association. The disease damages the body by injuring and weakening blood vessels, which increases the risk of heart attack, stroke, heart failure, kidney failure, and other circulatory system complications.

Eating well, maintaining a healthy weight, and physical activity can all help people control high blood pressure. The Heart Association recommends that people get their physician's permission to follow the government's guidelines for aerobic and strength training exercises.

Often physicians will recommend that only people who have their blood pressure under control participate in strenuous strength training workouts to avoid causing blood pressure spikes. They are also advised not to hold their breath when exerting themselves or lifting heavy weights over their heads. Both actions will elevate their blood pressure.

Useful Resource: American Heart Association at www.heart.org

6. Obesity

One in three Americans is obese and another third are categorized as overweight. The condition is becoming so great a threat to public health that the American Medical Association defined obesity as a disease in 2013. People who are obese are at greater risk of heart disease, heart failure, high blood pressure, cancer, diabetes, stroke, arthritis, and depression.

Eating a healthy diet is the most critical factor in weight loss. Regular exercise plays a secondary role that is more important for keeping lost weight off and promoting overall fitness and health. In some cases, health professionals will recommend medical intervention, including treatment with pharmaceuticals and surgery, to help obese people to lose weight. In addition, intensive counseling and assistance from a registered dietician are helpful in changing poor eating habits.

Obese people are encouraged to seek their physician's permission to follow the government's aerobic and strength training exercise guidelines. When considering aerobic exercises, obese people should focus on activities that will not exacerbate any pre-existing conditions. For example, low impact aerobic activities will be better for their ankles, knees and hips than high-impact activities. Obese people should also consider focusing their strength training efforts on using dumbbells, since they offer the widest range of motion without the potential tight fit or weight capacity limits posed by many gym machines. Note: The total weight capacity of exercise equipment must include the person's body weight and the amount of added weight they intend to lift on the machine.

Useful Resource: Obesity Society at Obesity.org

7. Osteoporosis

Osteoporosis, a disease defined by loss of bone mass, disproportionately affects women over the age of 50. Menopause, a poor diet that lacks calcium and vitamin D, inactivity, smoking, and drinking too much alcohol are all risk factors. People with osteoporosis have a greater risk of breaking their hips, spines and other bones.

The National Osteoporosis Foundation recommends that people with osteoporosis consume a healthy diet rich in fruits, vegetables, and foods that contain calcium and vitamin D. The foundation also recommends that they ask their physicians about appropriate weight-bearing and muscle-strengthening exercises to maintain and build bone density.

Those who have broken a bone or are at great risk for breaking bones are usually advised to avoid high-impact weight-bearing exercises, such as step aerobics, running, and tennis. Instead, they should participate in low-impact activities, such as brisk walking or using a stationary bike or elliptical machines. Strength training is usually okay, as long as the participant avoids positions that may result in broken bones. For example, some people with osteoporosis can break a bone in the spine by bending forward with an arched back.

The foundation recommends that people work with a physical therapist to decide which exercises to include in their fitness program.

Useful Resource: National Osteoporosis Foundation at NOF.org

8. Visual Impairment

People with impaired vision can often, with their physician's and opthamologist's approval, participate in many of the same aerobic and strength training exercises as non-impaired individuals. They may, however, need to exercise with a non-impaired trainer or buddy who can assist them through a course during aerobic exercise or around exercise machines and equipment during strength training sessions.

Some people with visual impairments need to choose exercises that will not exacerbate their condition. For example, people with diabetic retinopathy have to avoid exercises that will cause their blood pressure to spike or those that involve sudden movement that can cause further damage to their eyes.

In addition to improving their overall health, exercise gives visually impaired people an opportunity to socialize, which helps prevent depression.

Useful Resource: American Foundation for the Blind at AFB.org

FINAL THOUGHTS

Regardless of their physical challenges, the vast majority of people will greatly benefit from a carefully designed and implemented fitness program. It may take more time and effort to implement but the rewards, in terms of improved health and greater strength and mobility, will more than make up for the investment.

Lawrence S. Richardson, Jr.

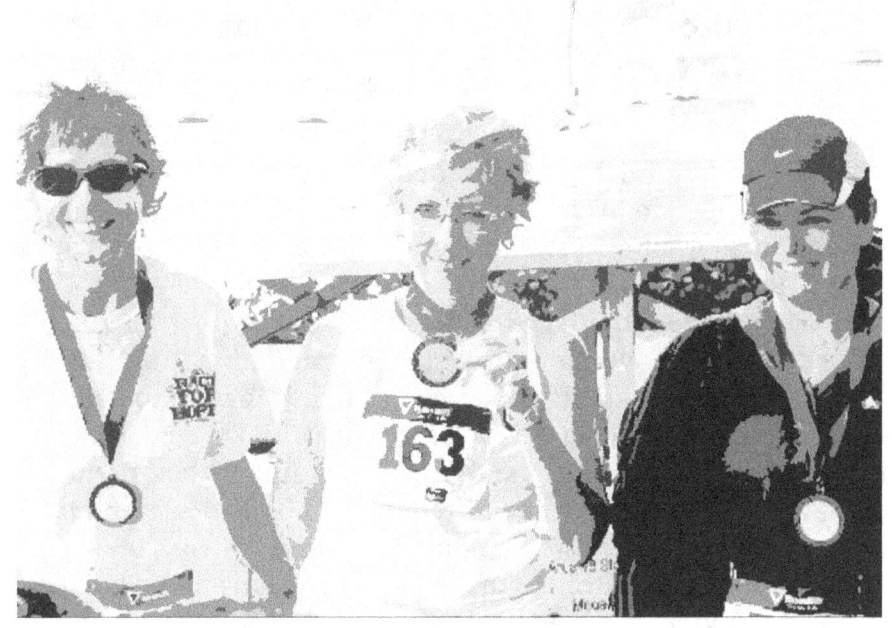

8 FIT BODY FIT MIND FOR LIFE!

Congratulations on making it to the final chapter of **Fit Body Fit Mind: Your Practical Guide to Aging Well!** You now possess the essential information you need to improve your health and age well through aerobic exercise, strength training, a healthy diet, and brain boosting activities. You have to admit it's pretty amazing that you can live a more fulfilling life using such basic techniques, but you can.

How do I know this? I have used the principles shared in this book for years. I'm rarely ill or injured, and I get the most enjoyment possible out of each and every day. To give you an idea of how to implement the Fit Body Fit Mind approach to health and well-being in your own life, I'll share my schedule with you.

Each week, I spend three alternate days running five to eight miles. The distance I go depends on how I feel and the weather. The three days in between my aerobic workout days I strength train using the Intermediate Strength Training program in this book. I precede each workout with a five to ten minute warm-up session and finish with the Intermediate Stretching routine.

The recipes in this book are for meals I make and eat on a regular basis. All my meals and snacks are rich in fruits, vegetables, whole grains, non-fat dairy and, occasionally, lean meat, chicken, and fish. I practice casual portion control to make sure I don't overeat.

When I first adopted this lifestyle, years ago, it took some effort. I had to overcome the strong gravitational pull of my couch to hit the road or gym. I had to fight the urge to eat junk food, of which chocolate is a particular pitfall. And I had to stop passively watching the world go by and engage my mind with the activities that appear in the Brain Boosters chapter.

The effort to become more active, eat healthier, and engage my mind has paid off enormously. The strength, balance, mobility, and mental agility I've gained have given me the ability to take on nearly any challenge without being fatigued or overwhelmed. I'm confident that once you implement the recommendations in this book in your own life, you'll have a similar transformation.

The major points you have to keep in mind as you begin this adventure are:

> **Be good to your body.** It's your friend, and you need to treat it well. Challenge it, but don't push it beyond its ability, or you will eventually find its limits by getting injured.

> **Be mindful in all you do.** When working out, proper form and total control over your body are more important than the amount of resistance you use or the speed at which you walk, run, or swim. The sensible, gradual approach to exercise will yield positive results while reducing your risk of injury.

> **Listen to your body.** Your body will tell you, through pain and fatigue, when you're exercising incorrectly.

When it does, stop what you're doing and listen to it. Then decide if you need to stop exercising or modify or replace the exercise that's harming you. Powering through pain will knock you out of the fitness game for a longer period of time than if you had addressed the problem when it first appeared.

➢ **Be patient.** Fad diets and fad exercise programs that promise quick results never work over the long haul. Use the principles in this book to create an exercise program and healthy diet that that works for you, then patiently wait for it to produce the desired results. If you're diligent, they will come, and you'll be all the healthier for it.

➢ **Find ways to stay motivated.** Repeating the same exercise routine week in and week out is a drag for even the most dedicated athletes. Switch out your aerobic and strength training exercises, try new equipment, and learn new and fun activities, like dancing, to shake up your routine. Also, reward yourself for reaching milestones with new sports gear, a trip, or dinner at your favorite restaurant.

➢ **Have fun! Fit Body Fit Mind: Your Practical Guide to Aging Well** isn't about sacrifice, it's about bringing a new, healthier approach to your everyday life that will reward you with more fulfillment. Just as being inactive feeds on itself and creates a life filled with a fatigue, illness, and pain, being active will fill your life with vitality, health, and mobility. Being fit also makes people more positive, which attracts upbeat people to them. Once the fitness fire is started, the updraft in your life is impossible to stop.

➢ **Seize Opportunities.** The world is full of people who will tell you reasons you can't exercise, you can't eat well, you can't travel, you can't learn, you can't write, you can't sing, you can't paint, you can't, you can't, you can't. Stop listening to the naysayers and explore what you want to do and how to do it. Be a door opener for yourself and others and engage your world. Also, always be kind, supportive, and enthusiastic of others who want to adopt a program that promotes body and mind fitness. If we all join this march, the world will be a better place.

A FEW MORE PRACTICAL TIPS FOR AGING WELL

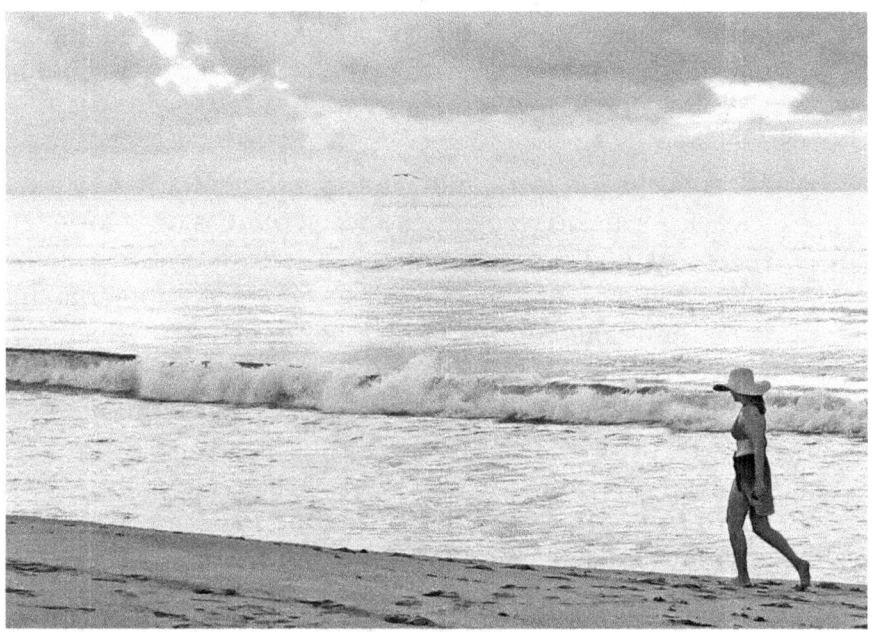

There are a few other practical tips not covered in the previous chapters that you can use today to improve your health and ability to age well:

> **Get the sleep you need**. Sleep is critical for recharging your body and mind. To ensure you get enough sleep, go to bed and wake up at the same time every day, create a dark, quiet room conducive to sleep, and avoid distractions that can alter your body clock – such as

televisions and computer screens – at least an hour before bed.

➢ **Take care of your teeth.** Research shows our mouths are breeding grounds for bacteria that can get into our bloodstream and promote the growth of artery-clogging plaques. For good oral health, brush at least twice a day for two minutes, floss once a day, and see your dentist every six months.

➢ **Take time out to de-stress.** The majority of Americans report heightened stress from their jobs and home life. Over a period of time, this can lead to high blood pressure and other health problems. It's important to take time each day to relax and bring calm to your system. How you do it is up to you. Some people find meditation works, while others reduce tension through aerobic and strength training exercise, stretching, or getting lost in a hobby they enjoy, such as reading, playing a musical instrument, or painting. Going out into Nature can also bring an enormous sense of peace.

➢ **Promote positive thoughts.** Arranging your life in a way that makes you generally happy will free you of the burden of negative thoughts so you can focus on the things that really matter, such as your health and well-being. Examine your life and see where you can replace situations and things that promote negativity with those that promote a positive outlook. You'll be amazed at how good life can be.

➢ **Always have something to look forward to on the short and long-terms.** One of the most basic ways to promote a healthy, positive outlook in life is to always have something to look forward to. It can be a visit with positive family and friends, a trip near or far, or beginning a fulfilling art project you've always dreamed of taking on. Whatever makes you happy, make sure to put it on your calendar so you have something to look forward to when times are tough.

➤ **Share your knowledge with others.** As you take on the Fit Body Fit Mind lifestyle, be sure to share your knowledge and experiences with others. Contributing to others' health and well-being will be rewarded many times over.

FINAL THOUGHTS

I've really enjoyed writing **Fit Body Fit Mind: Your Practical Guide to Aging Well.** I'm confident that if you apply the principles in this book, your life will improve.

I have one favor to ask of you. Please visit our companion website, Xeniors.com, and let me know how this basic approach to body and mind fitness and aging well is working for you and what you are doing differently to improve your own life that may help others.

If we build a large enough community, others may follow us by example and fit bodies and fit minds will become the norm instead of the exception, and more people will know the joys of aging well.

I look forward to seeing you there!